World Clinics

Dermatology

Atopic Dermatitis

World Clinics

Dermatology

Atopic Dermatitis

Editor-in-Chief
Rashmi Sarkar MD MNAMS

Guest Editor
Margarita Larralde MD PhD

June 2018 Volume 4 Number 1

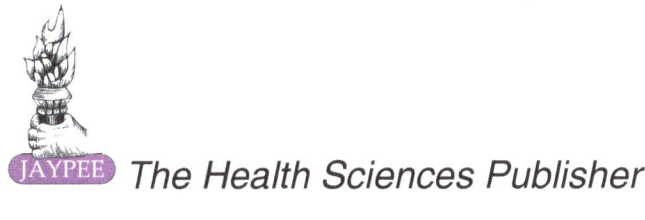

JAYPEE *The Health Sciences Publisher*

New Delhi | London | Panama

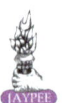 **Jaypee Brothers Medical Publishers (P) Ltd**

Headquarters

Jaypee Brothers Medical Publishers (P) Ltd
4838/24, Ansari Road, Daryaganj
New Delhi 110 002, India
Phone: +91-11-43574357
Fax: +91-11-43574314
Email: jaypee@jaypeebrothers.com

Overseas Offices

J.P. Medical Ltd
83 Victoria Street, London
SW1H 0HW (UK)
Phone: +44-2031708910
Fax: +02-03-0086180
Email: info@jpmedpub.com

Jaypee-Highlights Medical Publishers Inc
City of Knowledge, Bld. 235, 2nd Floor, Clayton
Panama City, Panama
Phone: +1 507-301-0496
Fax: +1 507-301-0499
Email: cservice@jphmedical.com

Jaypee Brothers Medical Publishers (P) Ltd
17/1-B Babar Road, Block-B, Shaymali
Mohammadpur, Dhaka-1207
Bangladesh
Mobile: +08801912003485
Email: jaypeedhaka@gmail.com

Jaypee Brothers Medical Publishers (P) Ltd
Bhotahity, Kathmandu, Nepal
Phone: +977-9741283608
Email: Kathmandu@jaypeebrothers.com

Website: www.jaypeebrothers.com
Website: www.jaypeedigital.com

Inquiries for bulk sales may be solicited at: jaypee@jaypeebrothers.com

This issue has been published in good faith that the contents provided by contributors contained herein are original, and is intended for educational purposes only. While every effort is made to ensure the accuracy of information, the publisher and the editors specifically disclaim any damage, liability, or loss incurred, directly or indirectly, from the use or application of any of the contents of this work. If not specifically stated, all figures and tables are courtesy of the contributing authors. Where appropriate, the readers should consult with a specialist or contact the manufacturer of the drug or device.

Cover images: (*Left*) Infantile atopic dermatitis. Dennie-Morgan fold below lower lids. Acute, oozing lesions on a background of erythema. *Courtesy:* Zubin K Mandlewala, Rashmi Sarkar. (*Middle*) Adult atopic dermatitis. Hyperpigmented, xerotic, lichenified anterior neck folds. *Courtesy:* Zubin K Mandlewala, Rashmi Sarkar. (*Right*) Testing antimicrobial susceptibility of *Staphylococcus aureus* using disc diffusion technique. *Courtesy:* Vanya Narayan, Rashmi Sarkar.

WORLD CLINICS DERMATOLOGY: Atopic Dermatitis

June 2018, Volume 4, Number 1

ISSN: 2347-7156

ISBN: 978-93-5270-355-5

Printed in India

Contributors

Editor-in-Chief

Rashmi Sarkar MD MNAMS
Professor
Department of Dermatology
Maulana Azad Medical College and Lok Nayak Hospital
New Delhi, India

Guest Editor

Margarita Larralde MD PhD
Chief
Department of Dermatology
Aleman Hospital
Department of Pediatric Dermatology
Ramos Mejía Hospital
Buenos Aires, Argentina

Contributing Authors

María E Abad MD
Staff
Department of Dermatology
Aleman Hospital
Department of Pediatric Dermatology
Ramos Mejía Hospital
Buenos Aires, Argentina

Pallavi Ailawadi MD DNB
Senior Resident
Department of Dermatology and STD
Maulana Azad Medical College and Associate Hospitals
New Delhi, India

Riti Bhatia MD
Senior Resident
Department of Dermatology and Venereology
All India Institute of Medical Sciences
New Delhi, India

Paula Boggio MD
Staff
Departments of Dermatology
Ramos Mejía Hospital and Pediatric Dermatology Hospital
Italiano de Buenos Aires
Buenos Aires, Argentina

Sandipan Dhar MD DNB FRCP
Professor and Head
Department of Pediatric Dermatology
Institute of Child Health
Kolkata, West Bengal, India

Vishal Gupta MD
Senior Research Associate
Department of Dermatology and Venereology
All India Institute of Medical Sciences
New Delhi, India

Akanksha Kaushik MD
Senior Resident
Department of Dermatology, Venereology, and Leprology
Postgraduate Institute of Medical Education and Research
Chandigarh, India

Paula C Luna MD
Staff
Department of Dermatology, Aleman Hospital
Department of Pediatric Dermatology
Ramos Mejía Hospital
Buenos Aires, Argentina

Rahul Mahajan MD
Assistant Professor
Department of Dermatology, Venereology, and Leprology
Postgraduate Institute of Medical Education and Research
Chandigarh, India

Zubin K Mandlewala DDV
Practicing Dermatologist, Reflectionz Clinic
Mumbai, Maharashtra, India

Isha Narang MD
Resident
Department of Dermatology, Venereology, and Leprology
Maulana Azad Medical College
New Delhi, India

Vanya Narayan MD DNB
Senior Resident
Department of Dermatology
Acharyashree Bhikshu Government Hospital
New Delhi, India

Indrashis Podder MD
RMO Cum Clinical Tutor
Department of Dermatology
College of Medicine and Sagore Dutta Hospital
Kolkata, West Bengal, India

Thomas Ruzicka MD
Head
Department of Dermatology and Allergology
Ludwig Maximilians University of Munich
Munich, Germany

Jaspriya Sandhu MD DNB
Senior Resident
Department of Dermatology, Venereology, and Leprology
Maulana Azad Medical College
New Delhi, India

Vinod K Sharma MD
Professor and Head
Department of Dermatology and Venereology
All India Institute of Medical Sciences
New Delhi, India

Sahana M Srinivas DNB DVD FRGUHS
Consultant
Department of Pediatric Dermatology
Indira Gandhi Institute of Child Health
Bangalore, Karnataka, India

Contents

World Clin Dermatol. 2018;4(1):xi.

Editorial

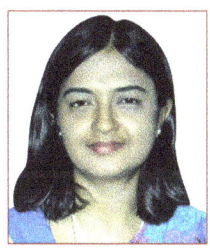

Rashmi Sarkar MD MNAMS
Editor-in-Chief

Atopic dermatitis in infants and children has been studied in details in the Western literature but there is lesser literature on this disease from the developing world. However, it remains a disease which significantly decreases the quality of life of the affected children as well as their parents and can remain a cause of loss of school days and economic burden.

Treatment is aimed at decreasing the dryness of the skin as well as to reduce the pruritus in the patients. Clinical manifestations of the disease can vary in different countries as also among children and adults. Recognition of minor features of the disease as well as atypical features are also important. Over several decades, the mainstay of treatment remains moisturizers, topical steroids, and topical calcineurin inhibitors. However, only recently, there is an excitement at the introduction of a phosphodiesterase inhibitor, crisabarole, a janus kinase inhibitor, tofacinib, and an FDA approved biological, dupilumab. Of course these still need to be evaluated over time.

However, one must also tactfully use age old treatment, combining it skillfully with newer advances to improve the life of the affected child. One also must give adequate information regarding general measures to be used in the child.

Rashmi Sarkar MD MNAMS
Professor, Department of Dermatology
Maulana Azad Medical College and Lok Nayak Hospital
New Delhi, India

Email: rashmisarkar@gmail.com

Abbreviations

AAP — American Academy of Pediatrics
ABCD — Airborne contact dermatitis
AD — Atopic dermatitis
AECs — Absolute eosinophil counts
AMPs — Antimicrobial peptides
APCs — Antigen presenting cells
APT — Atopy patch testing
AZA — Azathioprine
BSA — Body surface area
cAMP — Cyclic adenosine monophosphate
CI — Confidence interval
CLA+ — Cutaneous lymphocyte-associated antigen positive
CLRs — C-type lectin receptors
CoNS — Coagulase negative Staphylococcus
CRS — Raman microspectroscopy
CS — Contact sensitization
CSVA6 — Coxsackievirus A6
DARC — Danish Allergy Research Centre
DBPCFC — Double-blind placebo controlled food challenge
DCs — Dendritic cells
DDCs — Dermal dendritic cells
DNA — Deoxyribonucleic acid
EASI — Eczema Area Scoring Index
EC — Eczema coxsackium
ECP — Eosinophil cationic protein
FDA — Food and Drug Administration
FLG — Filaggrin
GM-CSF — Granulocyte-monocyte colony stimulating factor
hBD — Human β-defensins
HDM — House dust mite
HFMD — Hand, foot, and mouth disease
HIV — Human immunodeficiency virus

HOME — Harmonizing Outcomes Measures for Eczema
HSV — Herpes simplex virus
IDECs — Inflammatory dendritic epidermal cells
IFN-γ — Interferon gamma
IGA — Investigators' Global Assessment
IgE — Immunoglobulin E
Ig-FLCs — Ig-free light chains
IL — Interleukin
ILCs — Innate lymphoid cells
ISAAC — International Study of Asthma and Allergies in Childhood
ISAC — Immuno Solid-phase Allergen Chip
JAK — Janus kinases
KiGGS — German Health Interview and Examination Survey for Children and Adolescents
LDH — Lactate dehydrogenase
mDC — Myeloid DC
MMF — Mycophenolate mofetil
MPA — Mycophenolic acid
MRSA — Methicillin-resistant S. aureus
MTX — Methotrexate
NB-UVB — Narrowband ultraviolet B
NFAT — Nuclear factor of activated T cells
NK — Natural killer
NMFs — Natural moisturizing factors
NOD — Nucleotide-binding oligomerization domain-containing protein
OR — Odds ratio
PAMPs — Pathogen-associated molecular patterns
PBP — Penicillin-binding protein
PCRS — Pruritus Categorical Response Scale

pDC	Plasmacytoid DC	SPT	Skin prick test
PDE	Phosphodiesterase	STAT	Signal transducer and
PNRS	Pruritus Numerical-Rating		activator of transcription
	Scale	TARC	Thymus and activation-
POEM	Patient-Oriented Eczema		regulated chemokine
	Measurement	TB	Tuberculosis
PO-SCORAD	Patient oriented SCORAD	TC	Topical corticosteroids
POSTN	Periostin	TCI	Topical calcineurin
PRRs	Pattern recognition receptors		inhibitors
PVL	Panton-Valentine toxin	TCs	Topical corticosteroids
QOL	Quality of life	TEWL	Transepidermal water loss
RANTES	Regulated on activation,	Th2	T helper type 2
	normal T expressed and	TIS	Three Item Severity Score
	secreted	TLR	Toll-like receptor
RAST	Radioallergosorbent Test	TNF	Tumor necrosis factor
RCTs	Randomized control trials	TPMT	Thiopurine
SA-EASI	Self-assessed version of the		methyltransferase
	EASI	TSLP	Thymic stromal
SASSAD	Six Area, Six Sign Atopic		lymphopoietin
	Dermatitis	TSST-1	Toxic shock syndrome
SCCmec	Staphylococcal cassette		toxin-1
	chromosome mec	VAS	Visual Analogue Scale
SCORAD	Scoring Atopic Dermatitis	VISA	Vancomycin-intermediate
SD	Seborrheic dermatitis		*S. aureus*
SE	Staphylococcal enterotoxins	VRSA	Vancomycin-resistant
sIL-2R	Soluble interleukin-2		*S. aureus*
	receptor	WWT	Wet-wrap therapy

World Clin Dermatol. 2018;4(1):1-11.

Atopic Eczema—Epidemiology and Comorbidities

[1,*]Rahul Mahajan MD, [1]Akanksha Kaushik MD, [2]Thomas Ruzicka MD

[1]Department of Dermatology, Venereology, and Leprology
Postgraduate Institute of Medical Education and Research, Chandigarh, India
[2]Department of Dermatology and Allergology
Ludwig Maximilians University of Munich, Munich, Germany

ABSTRACT

Atopic dermatitis (AD), also called eczema, is a chronic inflammatory skin disease, with flares of acute pruritic lesions superimposed on underlying dry skin. The disease is often associated with other atopic conditions like allergic rhinitis, asthma, and food allergies and shows a global prevalence of up to 20% in children and up to 3% in adults. Recent evidence suggests AD to be a systemic disorder with significant systemic comorbidities. The artical provides a review of the current epidemiology and risk factors in AD, along with a brief discussion of associated comorbidities.

INTRODUCTION

Atopic dermatitis (AD) is a chronic relapsing inflammatory skin disease, characterized by episodes of acute pruritic lesions and an underlying dry skin. The epidemiology of AD is complex and ever-evolving. The disease usually begins in childhood, although onset has been reported to occur at any age. The nature of disease and its relapsing-remitting course is associated with significant morbidity, adversely affecting the quality of life in AD patients. This review aims to focus on the recent trends in epidemiology and the associated morbidity.

*Corresponding author
Email: drrahulpgi@yahoo.com

EPIDEMIOLOGY

Prevalence Studies

The onset of AD is mostly seen in children, although it can begin at any age.[1] Global prevalence is 15–20% in case of children and 1–3% in adults. In 30–50% patients, there is improvement in adolescence. Most worldwide data and trends regarding AD and other atopic disorders in children have been obtained via the International Study of Asthma and Allergies in Childhood (ISAAC), which has used a uniform validated methodology for comparing results in different pediatric population.[2]

In phase I of ISAAC study, the global prevalence varied between 3 and 20.5%.[3] Williams et al. compared the findings of ISAAC phase I versus ISAAC phase III and found that the prevalence of AD is increasing worldwide. In the 6–7 years group, there was overall rise in prevalence for AD in most centers. In the 13–14 years group, prevalence decreased in previously high-prevalence areas, including New Zealand and United Kingdom, whereas the prevalence increased in the developing countries.

International Study of Asthma and Allergies in Childhood phase III study reported the global variation in prevalence of AD to be highly variable across different countries, ranging from as low as 0.9% in India to as high as 22.5% in Ecuador in 6–7 years age group.[4] In 13–14 years age group, prevalence was similarly variable, ranging from 0.2% in China to 24.6% in Columbia. Highest prevalence in all age groups evaluated were found in Latin American countries and Africa. Active AD (current eczema) was higher in girls than boys.[5] In a systematic review by Deckers et al., AD prevalence in children was found to be more than 20% in developed countries, with rising trends in Africa, West and Northern Europe, and Eastern Asia.[6] The update on phase III ISAAC by Mallol et al. in 2013 has reported the global prevalence of AD to be 7.9% in the 6–7 years age group and 7.3% in 13–14 years age group. This update also established that the prevalence of AD is significantly higher in nonaffluent centers with low socioeconomic conditions.[7]

The previously held opinion that AD is an active disease only affecting children is no longer valid. Older studies have found prevalence of AD in adults ranging from 2.0 to 6.9%. Recent studies have suggested that AD may be more common in adults than previously thought. In the United States, the 1-year prevalence for AD in adults was found to be 10.2% in 2010 and 7.2% in 2012.[8] In the same 2012 study, peak prevalence was seen in early childhood (14%), decreased in adolescents (8%), and was stable in adults (6–8%). A study in Taiwan reported 8% prevalence of adult AD in a medical center.[9] A recent study in China has reported the prevalence of adult AD in outpatient department to be 4.6%. The same study suggested the onset age to be 35 years and the average age to be 40 years for adult AD.[10]

Regarding gender preference for AD, most studies suggest equal preponderance in males and females before 6 years of age.[11] Beyond 6 years of age, females are more commonly affected than males.[12,13]

Prevalence in India

Among Indian children studied in phase I of ISAAC study, the 12-month prevalence varied between 2.4 and 6%, with Kottayam in Kerala reporting more than 9% prevalence.[3] As per ISAAC phase III, the prevalence of current eczema as well as severe eczema in India in the age groups of 6–7 years as well as 13–14 years was below the global prevalence, being less than 5% at most centers.[4]

In a prospective hospital-based study from Bihar, the prevalence of AD was found to be 7.2% in children from 0 to 15-year age group, with male to female ratio being 1:1.3. Majority of patients (89.4%) had onset of AD before 5 years of age. Infantile AD had statistically significant higher Severity Scoring of Atopic Dermatitis (SCORAD) scores in all three grades of severity. The same study also reported significant increase in total serum immunoglobulin E (IgE) and absolute eosinophil count in 66% patients with AD.[14] Kumar et al. have reported 6.7% point-prevalence of AD in Indian patients across all four zones of India.[15] In a clinico-etiological study conducted in a tertiary health center in Gujarat, the prevalence of AD was found to be 4.3% in children.[16]

RISK FACTORS FOR DEVELOPMENT OF ATOPIC DERMATITIS

Hygiene Hypothesis

Studies have shown inverse relation of AD with overcrowding, large family size, and day care infections, whereas antibiotic use in early life has been suggested to be associated with greater risk of AD.[17] Observations like these have prompted further investigations into role of the so-called "hygiene hypothesis." This hypothesis suggests that with rising hygiene levels, there is reduced exposure to certain viral and bacterial pathogens in young life. Normally, microbial antigens induce anti-inflammatory cytokines like interleukin-10 and transforming growth factor-β. Deprivation of stimulation by microbes induces immune dysregulation and increases risk of sensitization in a genetically predisposed individual, thereby resulting in AD. In a recent cohort-based study, it was shown that antibiotic use within first 2 years of life is a risk factor for current AD, asthma, and allergic rhinitis in 5 year old children.[18] As reported in the recent German Health Interview and Examination Survey for Children and Adolescents (KIGGS) study, vaccination in first year of life was not associated with increased risk of AD.[19]

Birth Order

Many studies have reported that compared to second or higher birth order, first born children have a higher risk of developing AD and also that AD has inverse relationship with number of siblings in the family. An update on phase III of ISAAC study, as reported by Strachan et al., demonstrated inverse relation of "eczema ever" with increase in total number of siblings (p <0.0001). The inverse association with larger family size was significantly more in developed countries with high socioeconomic status.[20]

SMOKING

Environmental tobacco smoke exposure is one of the most important indoor air pollutants and has been evaluated in multiple studies. Lee et al. have reported association of childhood exposure to environmental tobacco smoke with adult-onset AD.[21] In a systematic review by Saulyte et al., allergic dermatitis was modestly associated with both active smoking and secondhand exposure to smoke, more in children and adolescents than adults.[22] In another recent systematic review and meta-analysis, Kantor et al. have concluded that both active and passive smoking exposure are associated with increased prevalence of AD in both children and adults.[23] Thyssen et al. have recently reported that the risk of major comorbidities is significantly increased in adult AD patients, especially smokers, as assessed by Charlson comorbidity index.[24]

Atopic March

Although AD can develop subsequent to appearance of other atopic lesions,[25] classically, it has often been said to precede the others, including food allergies, allergic rhinitis, and bronchial asthma.[26] This so-called "atopic march" is theorized to represent a sequential chain of epicutaneous sensitization by allergens, development of sensitized immune cells and their subsequent migration to respiratory epithelium.[27,28] Disruption of skin barrier and filaggrin mutations have been found to be consistently associated with atopic disorders. Patients with extrinsic AD (having specific IgE antibodies against environmental allergens) are found to be at higher risk for progressing in the atopic march to allergic rhinitis and asthma than those with intrinsic AD. The severity of AD directly correlates with risk of allergic rhinitis and with increased IgE antibodies.[29]

Breastfeeding and Other Dietary Influences

The effect of breastfeeding on the development of AD is still controversial. While some studies suggest protective effects of breastfeeding on AD,[30] others show insignificant or reverse effects.[31] The role of other dietary factors in AD is not clear. A systematic review has reported that a significant number of studies have reported the beneficial effects of fish oil supplementation during pregnancy as well as early childhood in reducing the prevalence of atopic disorders.[32] A recent study found no association between diet quality during pregnancy or in early life with AD or other atopic disorders in later life.[33]

Barrier Care with Prophylactic Emollients

Since impaired skin barrier has been hypothesized to have a key role in development of AD, recent focus has shifted to possible role of prophylactic use of emollients in preventing the development of AD. Simpson et al. reported statistically significant protective effect of daily full-dose emollient application against AD, in a randomized trial on 124 neonates.[34] Recently, the PEBBLES pilot study by Lowe et al. has reported significantly reduced incidence of AD and food allergies in infants treated with twice daily use of ceramide-dominant emollient.[35]

MORBIDITY IN ATOPIC DERMATITIS

Atopic dermatitis is associated with many complications and comorbidities. Atopic dermatitis has been proposed by some authors to be a systemic disease, with skin barrier disruption and immune dysregulation being pivotal in pathogenesis. Ocular disorders found to be associated with AD include allergic blepharoconjunctivitis, keratoconus, and posterior and anterior subcapsular cataracts. Gastrointestinal conditions found to be associated with AD include eosinophilic gastroenteritis and higher risk of inflammatory bowel disease, presumably related to Th2 cytokine pathway involvement as a common factor. Other associations like nephritic syndrome, neuropsychiatric illnesses, and metabolic syndrome have also been reported.[36]

Atopic Dermatitis and Infections

Altered cutaneous flora, with increased colonization by *Staphylococcus aureus* has been demonstrated.[37] The increased staphylococcal carriage produces superinfection of skin lesions in AD. Colonization with methicillin-resistant strains of *S. aureus* is also more common than methicillin-sensitive ones in these patients.[38,39] Studies have shown that *S. aureus* promotes Th2/Th22 inflammation in AD[40] and may even have a role in food allergies.[41] Patients with AD show higher risk for skin infection by herpes simplex virus, resulting in "eczema herpeticum."[42] Mathes et al. have reported increased infection by coxsackieviruses in AD, resulting in "eczema coxsackium."[43] Other infections like warts, streptococcal respiratory infections, urinary infections and otitis media have also been reported to be more prevalent in AD patients.[44]

Neuropsychiatric Morbidity

Itching in AD patients adversely affects the quality of life (QOL). Itching and emotional distress have a reinforcing effect on each other. While on one hand, itching produces increased mental stress and even suicidal tendency,[45] emotional stress itself has also been shown to result in increased itching.[46] Itching further results in sleep disturbances and daytime fatigue. Children with AD have a higher risk of learning and behavioral disorders like speech disorders and attention deficit hyperactivity disorder.[47] Even in adults, depression and anxiety disorders are more common in AD patients.[48,49] Recent studies have also reported increased odds of childhood nocturnal enuresis with allergic disorders, including AD.[50] A recent cross-sectional study in adolescents showed a significantly increased prevalence of migraine in AD.[51]

Cardiovascular Morbidity in Atopic Dermatitis

Recent studies have focused on the cardiovascular morbidity in AD patients. Obesity and increased waist circumference have been reported in children and adolescents with AD, as compared to controls.[52,53] Patients with AD have significant elevations in systolic as well as diastolic blood pressures in moderate to severe AD.[53] In a 2014 study by Su et al., AD was reported to be an independent risk factor for ischemic stroke in Taiwanese population.[54] However, some studies have reported that risk of cardiovascular disease and stroke is not increased in AD patients, when adjusted for factors like smoking, medication, and hypertension.[55,56] In a recent cross-sectional analysis from the Canadian Partnership for Tomorrow Project, AD was inversely associated with risk of myocardial infarction, stroke, hypertension, and type 2 diabetes mellitus.[57]

These findings suggest that rather than systemic inflammation, poor health behaviors, smoking, and medication related factors may be the major determinants of cardiovascular disease in AD patients.

Malignancy in Atopic Dermatitis

Many studies have focused on the relation between AD and malignancies. Chronic systemic inflammation, particularly shift from a Th1 type immunity to a Th2 type, as well as use of agents like cyclosporine in severe forms of AD have been postulated to play a role.[58,59] Arellano et al. have reported increased risk of cutaneous T cell lymphoma in AD, with risk more in severe forms.[60] Other studies have suggested that this association with lymphomas is overestimated and apparent association might be due to the misdiagnosis of cutaneous T cell lymphomas as AD.[61] Regarding other malignancies, recent studies and systematic reviews have shown inverse or no association between AD and risk of acute leukemia, actinic keratosis, basal cell carcinoma, malignant melanoma, and pancreatic and brain tumors.[62-64] Inverse association may be described by immune surveillance as well as IgE-mediated tumor antigen presentation by dendritic cells.[65]

Atopic Dermatitis and Autoimmunity

A connection between autoimmunity and AD has been suspected. Increased incidence of autoimmune disorders has been reported in atopic children. In a systematic review, Tang et al. reported a strong association between autoreactivity and AD.[66] Although IgE autoreactivity to various human proteins has been reported in AD patients,[67] further studies are needed to define the exact correlation in clinical terms.

Other Comorbidities

Patients with AD are prone to increased risk of fractures, on account of decreased bone mineral density.[68,69] This can be attributed to a variety of factors, including effects of cutaneous inflammation,[70] as well as widespread use of oral corticosteroids in treating even mild exacerbations, despite recommendations to the contrary.[71] Short stature has also been described more frequently in children with AD, with one older study putting prevalence in AD at 22%,[72] although later studies suggest that AD is not significantly associated with short stature.[73,74]

ECONOMIC IMPACT AND QUALITY OF LIFE IN ATOPIC DERMATITIS

In addition to direct health-related effects as described, AD also results in increased burden of costs, both direct and indirect, to the patient and family. Direct costs arise on account of medications, physician-visits, hospitalizations, as well as employing allergen-avoiding measures like dust and mite protectors. Indirect costs include absenteeism in school for children and loss of work hours for adult patients with AD.[75] An Indian study reported significantly high cost of care in AD, comparable to those with chronic diseases like diabetes mellitus.[76]

The QOL is adversely affected in all forms of AD across all ages. Mozaffari et al. have reported significant impact on QOL in both children and adult AD patients using the Dermatology Life Quality Index scores.[77] Holm et al. reported significant impact of AD on QOL in children, using an objective score called SCORAD.[78] Another study in AD patients between 4 and 70 years age demonstrated significantly inferior scores in AD patients on social functioning, vitality, and mental health subscales compared to the general population.[79] An international multicenter study has reported significant adverse impact on QOL and family QOL in children with AD.[80]

CONCLUSION

Atopic dermatitis represents a challenging disorder with epidemiological factors still not fully elucidated. The worldwide prevalence is rising with greater prevalence in affluent parts of the world. There is an inverse correlation with family size and birth order and role of environmental and dietary factors is increasingly being appreciated. Atopic dermatitis carries significant comorbidities in the form of infections and various systemic illnesses. Quality of life is significantly affected across all age groups and is an important consideration in deciding management.

Editor's Comment

Studies of disease prevalence of atopic dermatitis gives us an indication of its priority as a disease in that particular community. An increase in prevalence of this disease in the developing world also shows the role of environmental factors, and moving to a more westernized lifestyle. It is a disease with morbidity and decrease in quality of life of the patients, hence, emphasizing the need for newer therapeutic modalities.

Rashmi Sarkar

REFERENCES

1. Hanifin JM, Reed ML. A population-based survey of eczema prevalence in the United States. *Dermatitis.* 2007;18(2):82-91.
2. Nutten S. Atopic dermatitis: global epidemiology and risk factors. *Ann Nutr Metab.* 2015;66 Suppl 1:8-16.
3. Worldwide variation in prevalence of symptoms of asthma, allergic rhinoconjunctivitis, and atopic eczema: ISAAC. The International Study of Asthma and Allergies in Childhood (ISAAC) Steering Committee. *Lancet.* 1998;351(9111):1225-32.
4. Williams H, Stewart A, von Mutius E, et al. Is eczema really on the increase worldwide? *J Allergy Clin Immunol.* 2008;121(4):947-54 e15.
5. Odhiambo JA, Williams HC, Clayton TO, et al. Global variations in prevalence of eczema symptoms in children from ISAAC Phase Three. *J Allergy Clin Immunol.* 2009;124(6):1251-8.e23.
6. Deckers IA, McLean S, Linssen S, et al. Investigating international time trends in the incidence and prevalence of atopic eczema 1990-2010: A systematic review of epidemiological studies. *PLoS One.* 2012;7(7):e39803.
7. Mallol J, Crane J, von Mutius E, et al. The International Study of Asthma and Allergies in Childhood (ISAAC) Phase Three: A global synthesis. *Allergol Immunopathol (Madr).* 2013;41(2):73-85.

8. Silverberg JI. Public health burden and epidemiology of atopic dermatitis. *Dermatol Clin*. 2017;35(3):283-9.
9. Lan CC, Lee CH, Lu YW, et al. Prevalence of adult atopic dermatitis among nursing staff in a Taiwanese medical center: A pilot study on validation of diagnostic questionnaires. *J Am Acad Dermatol*. 2009;61(5):806-12.
10. Wang X, Shi XD, Li LF, et al. Prevalence and clinical features of adult atopic dermatitis in tertiary hospitals of China. *Medicine (Baltimore)*. 2017;96(11):e6317.
11. Verboom P, Hakkaart-Van L, Sturkenboom M, et al. The cost of atopic dermatitis in the Netherlands: An international comparison. *Br J Dermatol*. 2002;147(4):716-24.
12. Shamssain MH, Shamsian N. Prevalence and severity of asthma, rhinitis, and atopic eczema in 13- to 14-year-old schoolchildren from the northeast of England. *Ann Allergy Asthma Immunol*. 2001;86(4):428-32.
13. Grize L, Gassner M, Wuthrich B, et al. Trends in prevalence of asthma, allergic rhinitis and atopic dermatitis in 5-7-year old Swiss children from 1992 to 2001. *Allergy*. 2006;61(5):556-62.
14. Kumar MK, Singh PK, Patel PK. Clinico-immunological profile and their correlation with severity of atopic dermatitis in Eastern Indian children. *J Nat Sci Biol Med*. 2014;5(1):95-100.
15. Kumar S, Nayak CS, Padhi T, et al. Epidemiological pattern of psoriasis, vitiligo and atopic dermatitis in India: Hospital-based point prevalence. *Indian Dermatol Online J*. 2014;5(Suppl 1):S6-8.
16. Jawade SA, Chugh VS, Gohil SK, et al. A clinico-etiological study of dermatoses in pediatric age group in tertiary health care center in South Gujarat region. *Indian J Dermatol*. 2015;60(6):635.
17. Flohr C, Pascoe D, Williams HC. Atopic dermatitis and the 'hygiene hypothesis': Too clean to be true? Br J Dermatol. 2005;152(2):202-16.
18. Yamamoto-Hanada K, Yang L, Narita M, et al. Influence of antibiotic use in early childhood on asthma and allergic diseases at age 5. *Ann Allergy Asthma Immunol*. 2017;119(1):54-8.
19. Schlaud M, Schmitz R, Poethko-Muller C, et al. Vaccinations in the first year of life and risk of atopic disease - Results from the KiGGS study. *Vaccine*. 2017;35(38):5156-5162.
20. Strachan DP, Ait-Khaled N, Foliaki S, et al. Siblings, asthma, rhinoconjunctivitis and eczema: A worldwide perspective from the International Study of Asthma and Allergies in Childhood. *Clin Exp Allergy*. 2015;45(1):126-36.
21. Lee CH, Chuang HY, Hong CH, et al. Lifetime exposure to cigarette smoking and the development of adult-onset atopic dermatitis. *Br J Dermatol*. 2011;164(3):483-9.
22. Saulyte J, Regueira C, Montes-Martinez A, et al. Active or passive exposure to tobacco smoking and allergic rhinitis, allergic dermatitis, and food allergy in adults and children: A systematic review and meta-analysis. *PLoS Med*. 2014;11(3):e1001611.
23. Kantor R, Kim A, Thyssen JP, et al. Association of atopic dermatitis with smoking: A systematic review and meta-analysis. *J Am Acad Dermatol*. 2016;75(6):1119-25.e1.
24. Thyssen JP, Skov L, Hamann CR, et al. Assessment of major comorbidities in adults with atopic dermatitis using the Charlson comorbidity index. *J Am Acad Dermatol*. 2017;76(6):1088-92.e1.
25. Lowe AJ, Abramson MJ, Hosking CS, et al. The temporal sequence of allergic sensitization and onset of infantile eczema. *Clin Exp Allergy*. 2007;37(4):536-42.
26. Spergel JM, Paller AS. Atopic dermatitis and the atopic march. *J Allergy Clin Immunol*. 2003;112(6 Suppl):S118-27.
27. Dharmage SC, Lowe AJ, Matheson MC, et al. Atopic dermatitis and the atopic march revisited. *Allergy*. 2014;69(1):17-27.
28. Leung DY. New insights into atopic dermatitis: role of skin barrier and immune dysregulation. *Allergol Int*. 2013;62(2):151-61.
29. Bantz SK, Zhu Z, Zheng T. The atopic march: Progression from atopic dermatitis to allergic rhinitis and asthma. *J Clin Cell Immunol*. 2014;5(2). pii: 202.
30. Snijders BE, Thijs C, Dagnelie PC, et al. Breast-feeding duration and infant atopic manifestations, by maternal allergic status, in the first 2 years of life (KOALA study). *J Pediatr*. 2007;151(4):347-51, 51.e1-2.
31. Benn CS, Wohlfahrt J, Aaby P, et al. Breastfeeding and risk of atopic dermatitis, by parental history of allergy, during the first 18 months of life. *Am J Epidemiol*. 2004;160(3):217-23.

32. Kremmyda LS, Vlachava M, Noakes PS, et al. Atopy risk in infants and children in relation to early exposure to fish, oily fish, or long-chain omega-3 fatty acids: A systematic review. *Clin Rev Allergy Immunol.* 2011;41(1):36-66.

33. Nguyen AN, Elbert NJ, Pasmans S, et al. Diet quality throughout early life in relation to allergic sensitization and atopic diseases in childhood. *Nutrients.* 2017;9(8).). pii: E841.

34. Simpson EL, Chalmers JR, Hanifin JM, et al. Emollient enhancement of the skin barrier from birth offers effective atopic dermatitis prevention. *J Allergy Clin Immunol.* 2014;134(4):818-23.

35. Lowe AJ, Su JC, Allen KJ, et al. A randomised trial of a barrier lipid replacement strategy for the prevention of atopic dermatitis and allergic sensitization: The PEBBLES pilot study. *Br J Dermatol.* 2017. [Epub ahead of print].

36. Darlenski R, Kazandjieva J, Hristakieva E, et al. Atopic dermatitis as a systemic disease. *Clin Dermatol.* 2014;32(3):409-13.

37. Malajian D, Guttman-Yassky E. New pathogenic and therapeutic paradigms in atopic dermatitis. *Cytokine.* 2015;73(2):311-8.

38. Warner JA, McGirt LY, Beck LA. Biomarkers of Th2 polarity are predictive of staphylococcal colonization in subjects with atopic dermatitis. *Br J Dermatol.* 2009;160(1):183-5.

39. Lo WT, Wang SR, Tseng MH, et al. Comparative molecular analysis of meticillin-resistant Staphylococcus aureus isolates from children with atopic dermatitis and healthy subjects in Taiwan. *Br J Dermatol.* 2010;162(5):1110-6.

40. Brandt EB, Sivaprasad U. Th2 cytokines and atopic dermatitis. *J Clin Cell Immunol.* 2011;2(3).

41. Jones AL, Curran-Everett D, Leung DY. Food allergy is associated with Staphylococcus aureus colonization in children with atopic dermatitis. *J Allergy Clin Immunol.* 2016;137(4):1247-8.e1-3.

42. Beck LA, Boguniewicz M, Hata T, et al. Phenotype of atopic dermatitis subjects with a history of eczema herpeticum. *J Allergy Clin Immunol.* 2009;124(2):260-9, 9.e1-7.

43. Mathes EF, Oza V, Frieden IJ, et al. "Eczema coxsackium" and unusual cutaneous findings in an enterovirus outbreak. *Pediatrics.* 2013;132(1):e149-57.

44. Silverberg JI, Silverberg NB. Childhood atopic dermatitis and warts are associated with increased risk of infection: A US population-based study. *J Allergy Clin Immunol.* 2014;133(4):1041-7.

45. Halvorsen JA, Lien L, Dalgard F, et al. Suicidal ideation, mental health problems, and social function in adolescents with eczema: a population-based study. *J Invest Dermatol.* 2014;134(7):1847-54.

46. Langenbruch A, Radtke M, Franzke N, et al. Quality of health care of atopic eczema in Germany: Results of the national health care study AtopicHealth. *J Eur Acad Dermatol Venereol.* 2014;28(6):719-26.

47. Strom MA, Fishbein AB, Paller AS, et al. Association between atopic dermatitis and attention deficit hyperactivity disorder in U.S. children and adults. *Br J Dermatol.* 2016;175(5):920-9.

48. Dalgard FJ, Gieler U, Tomas-Aragones L, et al. The psychological burden of skin diseases: A cross-sectional multicenter study among dermatological out-patients in 13 European countries. *J Invest Dermatol.* 2015;135(4):984-91.

49. Yu SH, Silverberg JI. Association between atopic dermatitis and depression in US adults. *J Invest Dermatol.* 2015;135(12):3183-6.

50. Tsai JD, Chen HJ, Ku MS, et al. Association between allergic disease, sleep-disordered breathing, and childhood nocturnal enuresis: A population-based case-control study. *Pediatr Nephrol.* 2017;32(12):2293-301.

51. Shreberk-Hassidim R, Hassidim A, Gronovich Y, et al. Atopic dermatitis in Israeli adolescents from 1998 to 2013: Trends in time and association with migraine. *Pediatr Dermatol.* 2017;34(3):247-52.

52. Silverberg JI, Simpson EL. Association between obesity and eczema prevalence, severity and poorer health in US adolescents. *Dermatitis.* 2014;25(4):172-81.

53. Silverberg JI, Becker L, Kwasny M, et al. Central obesity and high blood pressure in pediatric patients with atopic dermatitis. *JAMA Dermatol.* 2015;151(2):144-52.

54. Su VY, Chen TJ, Yeh CM, et al. Atopic dermatitis and risk of ischemic stroke: A nationwide population-based study. *Ann Med.* 2014;46(2):84-9.

55. Andersen YM, Egeberg A, Gislason GH, et al. Risk of myocardial infarction, ischemic stroke, and cardiovascular death in patients with atopic dermatitis. *J Allergy Clin Immunol.* 2016;138(1):310-2 e3.

56. Drucker AM, Li WQ, Cho E, et al. Atopic dermatitis is not independently associated with nonfatal myocardial infarction or stroke among US women. *Allergy*. 2016;71(10):1496-500.

57. Drucker AM, Qureshi AA, Dummer TJ, et al. Atopic dermatitis and risk of hypertension, type-2 diabetes, myocardial infarction and stroke in a cross-sectional analysis from the Canadian Partnership for Tomorrow Project. *Br J Dermatol*. 2017;177(4):1043-51.

58. Josephs DH, Spicer JF, Corrigan CJ, et al. Epidemiological associations of allergy, IgE and cancer. *Clin Exp Allergy*. 2013;43(10):1110-23.

59. Chockalingam R, Downing C, Tyring SK. Cutaneous squamous cell carcinomas in organ transplant recipients. *J Clin Med*. 2015;4(6):1229-39.

60. Arellano FM, Wentworth CE, Arana A, et al. Risk of lymphoma following exposure to calcineurin inhibitors and topical steroids in patients with atopic dermatitis. *J Invest Dermatol*. 2007;127(4):808-16.

61. Tennis P, Gelfand JM, Rothman KJ. Evaluation of cancer risk related to atopic dermatitis and use of topical calcineurin inhibitors. *Br J Dermatol*. 2011;165(3):465-73.

62. Linabery AM, Jurek AM, Duval S, et al. The association between atopy and childhood/adolescent leukemia: A meta-analysis. *Am J Epidemiol*. 2010;171(7):749-64.

63. Deckert S, Kopkow C, Schmitt J. Nonallergic comorbidities of atopic eczema: An overview of systematic reviews. *Allergy*. 2014;69(1):37-45.

64. Schafer I, Mohr P, Zander N, et al. Association of atopy and tentative diagnosis of skin cancer - results from occupational skin cancer screenings. *J Eur Acad Dermatol Venereol*. 2017. [Epub ahead of print].

65. Platzer B, Elpek KG, Cremasco V, et al. IgE/FcεRI-mediated antigen cross-presentation by dendritic cells enhances anti-tumor immune responses. *Cell Rep*. 2015;pii:S2211-1247(15)00143-6.

66. Tang TS, Bieber T, Williams HC. Does "autoreactivity" play a role in atopic dermatitis? *J Allergy Clin Immunol*. 2012;129(5):1209-15.e2.

67. Mittermann I, Aichberger KJ, Bunder R, et al. Autoimmunity and atopic dermatitis. *Curr Opin Allergy Clin Immunol*. 2004;4(5):367-71.

68. Silverberg JI. Association between childhood atopic dermatitis, malnutrition, and low bone mineral density: A US population-based study. *Pediatr Allergy Immunol*. 2015;26(1):54-61.

69. Garg N, Silverberg JI. Association between eczema and increased fracture and bone or joint injury in adults: A US population-based study. *JAMA Dermatology*. 2015;151(1):33-41.

70. Uluckan O, Jimenez M, Karbach S, et al. Chronic skin inflammation leads to bone loss by IL-17-mediated inhibition of Wnt signaling in osteoblasts. *Sci Transl Med*. 2016;8(330):330ra37.

71. Sidbury R, Davis DM, Cohen DE, et al. Guidelines of care for the management of atopic dermatitis: Section 3. Management and treatment with phototherapy and systemic agents. *J Am Acad Dermatol*. 2014;71(2):327-49.

72. David TJ. Short stature in children with atopic eczema. *Acta Derm Venereol Suppl (Stockh)*. 1989;144:41-4.

73. Patel L, Clayton PE, Jenney ME, et al. Adult height in patients with childhood onset atopic dermatitis. *Arch Dis Child*. 1997;76(6):505-8.

74. Park MK, Park KY, Li K, et al. The short stature in atopic dermatitis patients: Are atopic children really small for their age? *Ann Dermatol*. 2013;25(1):23-7.

75. Sidbury R, Khorsand K. Evolving concepts in atopic dermatitis. *Curr Allergy Asthma Rep*. 2017;17(7):42.

76. Handa S, Jain N, Narang T. Cost of care of atopic dermatitis in India. *Indian J Dermatol*. 2015;60(2): 213.

77. Mozaffari H, Pourpak Z, Pourseyed S, et al. Quality of life in atopic dermatitis patients. *J Microbiol Immunol Infect*. 2007;40(3):260-4.

78. Holm EA, Wulf HC, Stegmann H, et al. Life quality assessment among patients with atopic eczema. *Br J Dermatol*. 2006;154(4):719-25.

79. Kiebert G, Sorensen SV, Revicki D, et al. Atopic dermatitis is associated with a decrement in health-related quality of life. *Int J Dermatol*. 2002;41(3):151-8.

80. Chernyshov PV, Jirakova A, Ho RC, et al. An international multicenter study on quality of life and family quality of life in children with atopic dermatitis. *Indian J Dermatol Venereol Leprol*. 2013;79(1):52-8.

World Clin Dermatol. 2018;4(1):12-9.

Etiopathogenesis of Atopic Dermatitis

[1]Indrashis Podder MD, [2,]*Rashmi Sarkar MD MNAMS

[1]Department of Dermatology, College of Medicine and Sagore Dutta Hospital
Kolkata, West Bengal, India
[2]Department of Dermatology, Maulana Azad Medical College and
Lok Nayak Hospital, New Delhi, India

ABSTRACT

Atopic dermatitis (AD) is one of the most common allergic inflammatory skin disorders usually affecting the pediatric population. It is a chronic, pruritic skin condition, demonstrating a frequently relapsing course. The etiopathogenesis of AD involves complex interplay of genetic, immunological and environmental factors including allergens, irritants, and microbial antigens resulting in skin barrier dysfunction, the hallmark pathological disturbance of this condition. Although the exact pathogenesis is still unclear, newer insights are being gained with each passing day. The recent developments in this aspect are discussed in this article to provide a comprehensive understanding of this subject.

INTRODUCTION

Atopic dermatitis is an inherited skin disorder characterized by the development of pruritic and eczematous lesions in a typical distribution (usually flexural folds) usually affecting the pediatric population.[1] It typically follows a chronic course interspersed with acute and frequent flare-ups and exacerbations. The pathogenesis of this disorder is complex, involving different genetic, immunological, and environmental factors (allergens and microbial antigens). Interaction of these factors result in epidermal barrier dysfunction and immune dysregulation—the two major pathological aberrations of this condition. Recently, new knowledge has been gained regarding these pathological interactions. The etiopathogenesis of AD has been discussed here along with the recent updates and relevant review of literature.

*Corresponding author
Email: rashmisarkar@gmail.com

ETIOPATHOGENESIS

Atopic dermatitis occurs as the result of complex interaction between different genetic, environmental, and immunologic factors. All these factors and the possible interplay between them have been discussed here briefly.

Genetic Factors

Genetic factors play an integral role in the pathogenesis of this disorder, characterized by the mutation of several genes. Increased genetic susceptibility is suggested by familial clustering of cases, concordance in monozygotic twins, but discordance in dizygotic twins and some recent reports of transmission of AD following bone marrow transplantation.[1] Most of the implicated genes have been found to regulate epidermal differentiation and immune system functioning. Some of the important genes and their details have been tabulated in table 1.[1-4]

Among all these genes, *FLG* gene mutation resulting in epidermal barrier dysfunction is most consistent, present in majority of the patients suffering from AD. However, recently skin barrier dysfunction due to deficiency of filaggrin has been recorded in a subset of European Caucasian patients although FLG gene is intact. This paradox may be explained by deoxyribonucleic acid methylation state or other variations of this gene, instead of the more common loss-of-function mutation.[2]

Immunological Factors

Dysregulation of immune system plays a major role in the etiopathogenesis of AD. The role of immune system may be discussed under the following subheadings.

Role of Innate Immunity

Innate immunity refers to the primordial and nonspecific immunity present in an individual since birth. In AD, the pattern recognition receptors present on the skin cells (monocytes, macrophages, and dendritic cells) show altered expression and function primarily due to genetic modification but also due to altered cytokine and chemokine profiles.[5,6] Toll-like receptor (TLR)-2 and -4 have been found to be the most important pattern recognition receptors in this regard.[2] Toll-like receptor signaling also regulates the epidermal barrier function apart from host defense mechanism. Interestingly, increased activation of TLR-2 and deficiency of TLR-4 have been recorded in mouse models with more severe forms of AD in recent studies.[7,8]

Table 1: Role of Genetic Factors in Etiopathogenesis of Atopic Dermatitis

Gene affected	Chromo-some	Protein/normal function	Result of genetic involvement
FLG	1q21	Filaggrin/maintaining epidermal barrier	Epidermal barrier dysfunction due to reduced filaggrin generation (loss-of-function mutation), the component responsible for binding keratin and maintaining the integrity of skin barrier
IFNG, IFNGR1	–	Interferon-γ and its receptor	Reduced expression of interferon-γ and its receptor (potent Th1 cytokine) resulting in increased susceptibility of skin infections particularly eczema herpeticum (disseminated HSV infection in AD patients)
NOD1, NOD2, DUSP1, ADM	–	Apoptosis related genes	Increased apoptosis of keratinocytes resulting in epidermal barrier dysfunction
ADAM17	–	Epidermal notch signaling proteins	Deletion mutation results in decreased epidermal notch signaling triggering activation of Th2 and/or Th17 pathway mediated aggravation of AD
CCDC109B, CCL5, CCL8, IFI35, LYN, RAB31, IFITM1, IFITM2	–	Genes regulating epidermal differentiation and functioning of immune system	Overexpression of these genes result in epidermal barrier dysfunction and immune system dysregulation
Genes coding for *IL-4, -5* and *-13; RANTES*	–	Immune system functioning	Immune system dysregulation
Genes encoding *TLR 2* and *TLR 9*	–	Innate immunity receptors	Immune system dysregulation
IgEFIgE FcεRI (high affinity IgE receptor)	–	IgE receptor	Increased sensitivity to IgE

HSV, herpes simplex virus; AD, atopic dermatitis; IgE, immunoglobulin E.

Role of Acquired Immunity

Abnormalities of acquired immunity plays a major role in the pathogenesis of this disorder. The lesional skin demonstrates increased infiltration of several immune cells like epidermal Langerhans' cells, inflammatory dendritic epidermal cells (IDECs), dermal dendritic cells (DDCs), monocytes, mast cells, neutrophils, basophils, eosinophils, innate lymphoid cells (ILCs), natural killer cells, fibroblasts, and various subsets of the T-cells.[2,9]

Among all these skin immune cells, epidermal Langerhans' cells and dermal dendritic cells play the pivotal role in causing this disorder.[1] Both these cells are antigen presenting cells (APCs) and they are activated when antigens bind to them. Circulating T-cells which express cutaneous lymphocyte-associated antigen home to the skin where they are further primed by these activated APCs.[2] The primed T-cells then secrete several inflammatory cytokines and chemokines, notably interleukin (IL)-4 and IL-13 to activate the T helper type 2 (Th2) pathway. These cytokines also reduce filaggrin expression and increase IgE synthesis, thus weakening the epidermal barrier and enhancing allergic sensitivity.[2] Recent studies have demonstrated that epidermal and dermal DCs in AD show increased expression of high affinity IgE receptors on their surface, which is a hallmark feature of this condition.[10]

Monocytes also play an important role by being differentiated into macrophages and dendritic cells in an inflammatory mileu. These dendritic cells present the antigen to T-cells in the draining lymph nodes. Recent studies have shown that monocytes in AD show reduced tumor necrosis factor (TNF)-β signaling[11] and impaired interferon-γ responsiveness,[12] thus stimulating the Th2 immunological pathway (as both Th1 cytokines are downregulated).

Mast cells have also been implicated in the pathogenesis of AD as lesional skin shows increased number of mast cells. Mast cells secrete both IL-31[13] and histamine,[14] which promote inflammation in these patients. However, the role of basophils is still unclear.[2]

Recently, ILCs have been observed to worsen AD by generating Th2 type cytokines notably IL-5, IL-9, and IL-13 to promote local inflammation after antigenic stimulation.[15]

Although Th2 immunological pathway plays the major role in acute stage of AD, its chronic phase is mediated by Th0 (features of both Th1 and Th2) and Th1 pathways.[1] The major Th2 cytokines are IL-4, IL-5, and IL-13; secreted by the activated T-cells. The roles of these cytokines are given below:

- Reduced synthesis of filaggrin (IL-4, IL-13), thus leading to epidermal barrier dysfunction. Besides, these Th2 mediators also cause skin barrier dysfunction by increasing the level of serine protease kallikrein 7 in the epidermis
- Enhanced synthesis of IgE (Ig switch) resulting in heightened sensitivity to allergens (IL-4, IL-13)
- Interleukin-4 stimulates mast cells to secrete inflammatory mediators like histamine
- Interleukin-5 is responsible for development and survival of eosinophils; these cells predominate in the subacute stage.

The switch from Th2 to Th0/1 pathway is mediated by cytokines like IL-12 and IL-18, which are secreted by the IDECs.[1] Chronic AD also shows increased level of Th22 cells which secrete IL-22, responsible for arresting terminal differentiation and inducing epidermal hyperplasia.[1] Th17 cells are also elevated in acute AD, but less marked than psoriasis; although their role in AD is still not clear.[16] Interleukin-25, an important member of the IL-17 family, also promotes AD by activating Th2 pathway and the DDCs. Furthermore, IL-25 also reduces filaggrin synthesis in the keratinocytes.[2]

Another important chemical mediator which deserves mention is thymic stromal lymphopoietin produced by the keratinocytes under the influence of TNF-α and other Th2 cytokines (IL-4, IL-13, and IL-31). Thymic stromal lymphopoietin acts in conjunction with IL-33 (another tissue derived cytokine) to promote Th2 mediated inflammation. Thymic stromal lymphopoietin also facilitates the switch to Th0/1 pathway.[1]

Tumor necrosis factor-α, a Th1 cytokine, also plays an important role in AD by reducing the synthesis of epidermal lipids like free fatty acids and ceramides. Additionally, TNF-α along with TNF-like weak inducer of apoptosis leads to keratinocyte apoptosis resulting in the skin lesions of AD.[17] Recent studies have deciphered the role of some chemokines like CCL17 and CCL22 in AD by increasing the infiltration of DCs and T-lymphocytes in the lesional skin.[18]

Environmental Factors

Several environmental factors have been implicated to play a role in the pathogenesis of this disease, some of the important ones are briefly discussed below.

Infections

Infections probably play the most important role in the pathogenesis of AD. Several microbes enter through the skin and these microbial antigens interact with the immune system to facilitate the development of AD. Microbes can enter through the skin because of several reasons:[1,2]

- Weakened epidermal barrier function (reduced fialaggrin)—physical defect
- Increased skin pH which may allow greater adherence and multiplication of these microbes—chemical barrier defect
- Defects in the TLRs which hinder the proper recognition of microbial antigens, thus impeding immune response
- Elevated Th2 cytokines reduce the synthesis of antimicrobial peptides by keratinocytes notably LL-37 (cathelicidin) and β-defensins 2 and 3
- *Staphylococcus aureus,* a common microbial agent releases virulence factors like α-toxins and other protease inhibitors leading to apoptosis of the keratinocytes, thus further weakening the skin barrier
- *Staphylococcus aureus* also activates T-cells and enhances IgE hypersensitivity in a superantigen mediated pathway. These superantigens also cause a marked

depletion in steroid responsiveness of the T-cells, resulting in therapeutic difficulties.

All these factors predispose atopic individuals to widespread skin infections due to bacteria (*Staphylococcus aureus, Propionibacteria,* and *Corynebacteria*), viruses (herpes, molluscum, and vaccinia) and possibly dermatophytes and *Malassezia* yeasts. Recently, Penders et al.[19] have proposed the etiological role of gut microbiome (*Lactobacillus, Bacteroides,* and *Clostridia*) in addition to skin microbiome. The authors have suggested several risk factors which may increase gut microbial involvement like higher birth order, increased number of siblings, and lack of breastfeeding. However, the exact role of gut microbiomes is still not clear.

In a subset of AD patients, some factors like elevated serum level of IgE, mutations in the *IFNG* and *IFNGR1* genes and higher IL-25 expression may increase the risk of disseminated herpes infection called eczema herpeticum.[2]

External Allergens

Food allergens and aeroallergens have been implicated by some authors in the pathogenesis of atopic dermatitis; however, their role remains controversial. Among aeroallergens house-dust mite (*Dermatophagoides pteronyssinus*) and ragweed pollen allergens[2] are most important. All these allergens may trigger immune response following sensitization, which usually occurs around infancy. Recently, Dai et al.[20] have shown that these allergens activate inflammasomes in keratinocytes which may promote AD by the Th1 or Th17 pathways. Notably, inflammasomes are also activated by *S. aureus.*

Climate

Atopic dermatitis is exacerbated during winter and dry climate. So proper measures should be taken to prevent these flare-ups.

Stress

Kwon et al.[21] have suggested that degree of stress has a positive correlation with the development and severity of AD. Interestingly, educational level of parents is also associated with AD (higher level of education increases the severity).

CONCLUSION

Pathogenesis of AD is a complex phenomenon which involves the interplay of genetic, immunologic, and environmental factors. Further identification of these factors at the cellular and molecular levels would help to develop newer therapeutic modalities, which may help us to contain this chronic disorder.

Editor's Comment

The role of allergic factors, microbes and food in the causation of atopic dermatitis still remains an important factor in disease causation. Studies on the role of genetic factors, filaggrin mutations with geographical variability, and thymic stromal lymphopoietin are emerging areas of research. Besides skin microbial involvement, gut microbial involvement is also required.

Rashmi Sarkar

REFERENCES

1. Tom WL, Eichenfield LF. Eczematous disorders. In: Eichenfield LF, Frieden IJ, Zaenglein A, et al., editors. Neonatal and infant dermatology. 3rd ed. Elsevier Health Sciences; 2015. pp. 216-32.
2. Peng W, Novak N. Pathogenesis of atopic dermatitis. *Clin Exp Allergy.* 2015;45:566-74.
3. Leung DY, Gao PS, Grigoryev DN, et al. Human atopic dermatitis complicated by eczema herpeticum is associated with abnormalities in IFN-γ response. *J Allergy Clin Immunol.* 2011;127:965-73.
4. Franzke CW, Cobzaru C, Triantafyllopoulou A, et al. Epidermal ADAM17 maintains the skin barrier by regulating EGFR ligand-dependent terminal keratinocyte differentiation. *J Exp Med.* 2012;209:1105-19.
5. Novak N, Yu CF, Bussmann C, et al. Putative association of a TLR9 promoter polymorphism with atopic eczema. *Allergy.* 2007;62:766-72.
6. Hasannejad H, Takahashi R, Kimishima M, et al. Selective impairment of Toll-like receptor 2-mediated proinflammatory cytokine production by monocytes from patients with atopic dermatitis. *J Allergy Clin Immunol.* 2007;120:69-75.
7. Kaesler S, Volz T, Skabytska Y, et al. Toll-like receptor 2 ligands promote chronic atopic dermatitis through IL-4-mediated suppression of IL-10. *J Allergy Clin Immunol.* 2014;134:92-9.
8. Brandt EB, Gibson AM, Bass S, et al. Exacerbation of allergen-induced eczema in TLR4-and TRIF-deficient mice. *J Immunol.* 2013;191:3519-25.
9. Berroth A, Kühnl J, Kurschat N, et al. Role of fibroblasts in the pathogenesis of atopic dermatitis. *J Allergy Clin Immunol.* 2013;131:1547-54.
10. Novak N. An update on the role of human dendritic cells in patients with atopic dermatitis. *J Allergy Clin Immunol.* 2012;129:879-86.
11. Peng WM, Maintz L, Allam JP, et al. Attenuated TGF-β1 responsiveness of dendritic cells and their precursors in atopic dermatitis. *Eur J Immunol.* 2013;43:1374-82.
12. Gros E, Petzold S, Maintz L, et al. Reduced IFN-γ receptor expression and attenuated IFN-γ response by dendritic cells in patients with atopic dermatitis. *J Allergy Clin Immunol.* 2011;128:1015-21.
13. Otsuka A, Kabashima K. Mast cells and basophils in cutaneous immune responses. *Allergy.* 2015;70:131-40.
14. Novak N, Peng WM, Bieber T, et al. FcεRI stimulation promotes the differentiation of histamine receptor 1-expressing inflammatory macrophages. *Allergy.* 2013;68:454-61.
15. Salimi M, Barlow JL, Saunders SP, et al. A role for IL-25 and IL-33-driven type-2 innate lymphoid cells in atopic dermatitis. *J Exp Med.* 2013;210:2939-50.
16. Guttman-Yassky E, Nograles KE, Krueger JG. Contrasting pathogenesis of atopic dermatitis and psoriasis—Part I: Clinical and pathologic concepts. *J Allergy Clin Immunol.* 2011;127:1110-8.
17. Zimmermann M, Koreck A, Meyer N, et al. TNF-like weak inducer of apoptosis (TWEAK) and TNF-α cooperate in the induction of keratinocyte apoptosis. *J Allergy Clin Immunol.* 2011;127:200-7.

18. Gros E, Bussmann C, Bieber T, et al. Expression of chemokines and chemokine receptors in lesional and nonlesional upper skin of patients with atopic dermatitis. *J Allergy Clin Immunol.* 2009;124:753-60.
19. Penders J, Stobberingh EE, van den Brandt PA, et al. The role of the intestinal microbiota in the development of atopic disorders. *Allergy.* 2007;62:1223-36.
20. Dai X, Sayama K, Tohyama M, et al. Mite allergen is a danger signal for the skin via activation of inflammasome in keratinocytes. *J Allergy Clin Immunol.* 2011;127:806-14.
21. Kwon JA, Park EC, Lee M, et al. Does stress increase the risk of atopic dermatitis in adolescents? Results of the Korea Youth Risk Behavior Web-based Survey (KYRBWS-VI). *PloS One.* 2013;8:e67890.

World Clin Dermatol. 2018;4(1):20-5.

Skin Barrier in Atopic Dermatitis

*Paula C Luna MD, Margarita Larralde MD PhD

Department of Dermatology, Aleman Hospital; Department of Pediatric Dermatology
Ramos Mejía Hospital, Buenos Aires, Argentina

ABSTRACT

The skin is the largest organ in the body. One of its main functions is to act as a physical and chemical barrier. The stratum corneum, the upper most layer of the epidermis, is a brick and mortar-like structure, is the true responsible of this function. It is a complex unit and depends of multiple factors to function correctly. For that reason, barrier defects might be determined by a constellation of host and environmental factors. A defective skin barrier contributes to the pathogenesis of atopic dermatitis (AD). Filaggrin mutations, irregularities in other structural proteins, altered lipidic composition or proteolytic enzymes as well as malfunction of some factors of the innate immunity, can all compromise the skin barrier and have all been shown to be, on their own or in association with other defects, responsible of the altered skin barrier in AD.

This article provides a summary of the different components of the skin barrier and how they are altered in AD.

INTRODUCTION

Atopic dermatitis (AD) is the most common inflammatory skin disease affecting around 15–30% of children and 1–3% of adult population worldwide with a steady growth in incidence in the past decades. For many years, it was considered an "inside-out" disease, analogous to the intrinsic asthma—an immune-mediated disease with a reactive epidermal hyperplasia. More updated knowledge also hypothesizes on an "outside-in" theory, suggesting that epidermal-barrier alterations happen first, leading to a secondary immune activation.[1] Probably both hypothesis could sum up and have an integrated role in disease development[2] in genetically predisposed individuals exposed to certain environmental factors.

*Corresponding author
Email: paulacarolinaluna@gmail.com

One of the main functions of the skin is to act as a protective barrier against a variety of external stimuli, mainly irritants and allergens.[3] In order to achieve this in the outer part of the epidermis, keratinocytes lose their nucleus and become flat and together with the highly lipidic intercellular matrix form the stratum corneum.[4]

The scope of this article is to review the knowledge regarding the role of the "skin barrier" in the development and perpetuation of AD.

SKIN BARRIER

Among the many functions of the skin, protection and defense is probably one of the most important. This is achieved through the regulation of the transepidermal water loss (TEWL) as well as by being a physical barrier for chemical irritants and allergens and the first defense against microorganisms.

The stratum corneum in the outer layer of the epidermis and is the main component of the skin barrier. It is composed of mature keratinocytes (corneocytes), several important proteins (filaggrin and proteins of the tight junctions), as well as surface lipids forming the intercellular matrix.

COMPONENTS OF THE SKIN BARRIER

Corneocytes

Corneocytes are mature keratinocytes. Cornification is the name of the process by which keratinocytes evolve and mature from the basal layer to the outer epidermis. In this process, the cells lose its nuclei and organelles, and form a rigid envelope, becoming flat and arrange in an overlapping fashion.[5]

Filaggrin

Filaggrin (filament-aggregating protein) is an intracellular protein produced by the keratinocytes and stored as profilaggrin polymers in keratohyalin granules in the stratum granulosum. After dephosphorylation and proteolysis by serine proteases, profilaggrin converts into multiple monomers of filaggrin in the interface between stratum granulosum and the stratum corneum.[6] These monomers then bind to intermediate filaments making the stratum corneum stronger. As the water gradient in the outer layers of the epidermis decrease, proteases called natural moisturizing factors hydrolyse filaggrin into hygroscopic amino acids such as arginine, glutamine and their derivatives playing a major role in stratum corneum hydration and pH maintenance.[3]

Several genetic factors may alter the filaggrin gene (*FLG*) expression. The loss of function in the *FLG* has been described in ichthyosis vulgaris[3] and also is the most commonly associated genetic component with a risk of AD development, severity, and increased propensity toward other atopic conditions (respiratory hyperreactivity, allergies, peanut allergy, elevated IgE serum levels). It is also associated with an increased risk of early onset of the disease as well as persistence of AD in adulthood.[7,8]

Different *FLG* mutations have been described, with loss of function (null) mutations being the most frequent (in around 10–50% of AD cases). It has also been found in up to 9% of non-AD population. Patients with *FLG* mutations also may outgrow their disease or have extended remissions.

Filaggrin gene mutations are the strongest risk factor known to date for the development of AD. However, the role of *FLG* mutations in the altered skin barrier function in AD is inconclusive.[9]

Other Epidermal Proteins

Upper keratinocytes are firmly attached to each other by corneodesmosomes. These proteins have also been proved to be defective in AD. Several studies have demonstrated a reduced expression of corneodesmosin, desmocolin-1 and desmoglein-1, loricrin, and involucrin in AD.[10]

Th2-associates factors [such as interleukin (IL)-4, IL-13, and histamine] have also shown to decrease the expression of corneodemosomal and cornified envelope proteins. For these reasons, a relationship between the inflammation and the cornified envelope has been suggested.

Tight junctions also have a very important role in maintaining skin barrier. They are composed by claudin family proteins, occludins, tricellulin, zonula occludens, and junction adhesion molecules. In AD, different allergens and microorganisms such as *Staphylococcus spp.* might disrupt these tight junctions by downregulating some of these proteins. On the other hand, reduced levels of these proteins might also play a role in the susceptibility to staphylococcal and herpetic infection in AD patients.

Lipids

Lipids are crucial in the maintenance of the epidermal barrier function. They fill intercellular space with highly organized lipids with a characteristic composition and organization. The major lipid classes in the stratum corneum are ceramides, free fatty acids, and cholesterol.[9]

Lipid precursors and lipid-processing enzymes are released from the granules of the keratinocytes in the stratum granulosum. Glycosylceramides, sphingomyelin and phospholipids, are processed into ceramides, cholesterol, and free fatty acids. In healthy skin, ceramides constitute the predominant lipids.[11] Decreased levels of ceramides, altered ceramide composition, and a change in the ceramide:cholesterol ratio have also been demonstrated in AD, and are thought to be also responsible of an enhanced skin permeability.

Several inflammatory cytokines have been shown to alter the ceramide production with a reduction of expression with IL-4 and IL-6 and an increase with interferon-γ and tumor necrosis factor-α.[11] The increased expression of different lipid-processing enzymes (sphingomyelinase and sphingomyelinase deacyclase) and the novel expression of others (such as the glucosyceramide deacyclase) might also be responsible of the decrease in ceramide.

Some studies have shown that the level of long-chain ceramides is reduced and the level of very short chain ceramides is increased in nonlesional AD skin.

Apart from the lipid composition and organization, the lipid:protein ratio is also an important factor for the altered skin barrier function. The lipid:protein ratio has shown to correlate strongly with inverse TEWL values, and is significantly lower in both nonlesional and lesional stratum corneum of AD patients compared to healthy controls.[9]

Proteolytic Enzymes

Barrier desquamation is crucial for maintaining a normal structure and thickness of the skin,[12] its homeostasis is maintained by the balanced action of proteases and their inhibitors.

Proteases play a role in the degradation of the corneodesmosomes, the regulation of lipid-processing enzymes and antimicrobial peptides, as well as in every other process involved in the dynamic maturation of the skin and its balance (cytokine expression, inflammation, apoptosis, tissue repair, and chemotaxis).

Alteration in the proteases kallikreins, cathepsins, and caspase-14 have all been implicated to play a role in AD. Protease inhibitors, such as the protease inhibitor lymphoepithelial Kazal-type related inhibitor, which is mutated in Netherton syndrome patients, have also been implicated.[13]

Antimicrobial Peptides

Antimicrobial peptides (AMPs) are also a very important part of skin barrier homeostasis. These are cationic enzymes, produced mainly by keratinocytes, that target bacteria, fungi, and viruses by permeabilizing their outer membrane, resulting in microbial lysis, through interactions with anionic components. They also play a role in recruiting inflammatory cells stimulating the expression of cytokines and chemokines. When there is inflammation, these peptides are also produced by other cell types such as neutrophils and mast cells.

Of the several families of AMPs, human β-defensins (hBD) and cathelicidins are the most studied in the human skin.[14] Some of these are constitutively expressed and others are only induced by inflammation.

Their role in AD is not well elucidated due to its complexity. While some studies have shown a marked reduction in the expression of the cathelicidin LL-37 and the β-defensins 2 in AD skin compared with psoriatic skin, other studies have shown higher levels of AMPs in the skin of these patients when comparing lesional to nonlesional skin. Furthermore, cytokines also play a role in regulating this peptides with IL-4 and IL-13 having an inhibiting effect on the hBD-2 and -3 gene while the neutralization of these interleukins enhances the expression of hBD-2 and -3 and LL-37.[11,15]

CONCLUSION

Skin barrier function in AD patients is defective, as a result of reduced levels of lipids that form the stratum corneum, filaggrin or claudin defects, altered proteases, and trauma from constant scratching.[16] This barrier defect increases TEWL and reduces capacitance as well as increasing susceptibility to infection to both *Staphylococcus* and *Herpes simplex virus*.

For all these reasons, maintaining or restoring the skin barrier is of vital importance in the treatment of AD and is considered a pillar in the management of this condition. The constant evolution and study of the skin barrier physiology will allow us to evolve in the knowledge of this disease and develop strategies to better help our patients.

Editor's Comment

The role of the skin barrier in the start and perpetuation of atopic dermatitis (AD) remains central to the pathogenesis of AD. Most of the research on emollients, one of the mainstay in the treatment of atopic dermatitis is directed towards improving epidermal barrier function. Maintaining the integrity of the skin barrier under adverse conditions would be fundamental to the improvement of atopic dermatitis.

Rashmi Sarkar

REFERENCES

1. Czarnowicki T, Krueger JG, Guttman-Yassky E. Skin barrier and immune dysregulation in atopic dermatitis: An evolving story with important clinical implications. *J Allergy ClinImmunol Pract*. 2014:4;371-9 quiz 380-1.
2. Bieber T. Atopic dermatitis. *N Engl J Med*. 2008;358:1483-94.
3. Otsuka A, Nomura T, Rerknimitr P, et al. The interplay between genetic and environmental factors in the pathogenesis of atopic dermatitis. *Immunol Rev*. 2017;278:246-62.
4. Proksch E, Brandner JM, Jensen JM. The skin: An indispensable barrier. *Exp Dermatol*. 2008;17:1063-72.
5. Mancini AJ, Lawley LP. Structure and function of newborn skin. In: Neonatal and infant dermatology. Eichenfield L, Freiden I, editors. 3rd ed. Elsevier Saunders; 2015. pp. 14-23.
6. Zaniboni MC, Samorano LP, Orfali RL, et al. Skin barrier in atopic dermatitis: Beyond filaggrin. *An Bras Dermatol*. 2016;91:472-8.
7. an den Oord RA, Sheikh A. Filaggrin gene defects and risk of developing allergic sensitisation and allergic disorders: systematic review and meta-analysis. *BMJ*. 2009;b2433:339.
8. Rodriguez E, Baurecht H, Herberich E, et al. Meta-analysis of filaggrin polymorphisms in eczema and asthma: Robust risk factors in atopic disease. *J Allergy ClinImmunol*. 2009;123:1361-70.
9. Janssens M, van Smeden J, Puppels GJ, et al. Lipid to protein ratio plays an important role in the skin barrier function in patients with atopic eczema. *Br J Dermatol*. 2014;170:1248-55.
10. Guttman-Yassky E, Suarez-Farinas M, Chiricozzi A, et al. Broad defects in epidermal cornification in atopic dermatitis identified through genomic analysis. *J Allergy ClinImmunol*. 2009;124:1235-44.e58.
11. Agrawal R, Woodfolk JA. Skin barrier defects in atopic dermatitis. *Curr Allergy Asthma Rep*. 2014;14:433.
12. Wolf R, Wolf D. Abnormal epidermal barrier in the pathogenesis of atopic dermatitis. *Clin Dermatol*. 2012;30:329-34.
13. Chavanas S, Bodemer C, Rochat A, et al. Mutations in SPINK5, encoding a serine protease inhibitor, cause Netherton syndrome. *Nat Genet*. 2000;25:141-2.
14. Braff MH, Bardan A, Nizet V, et al. Cutaneous defense mechanisms by antimicrobial peptides. *J Invest Dermatol*. 2005;125:9-13.
15. Nomura I, Goleva E, Howell MD, et al. Cytokine milieu of atopic dermatitis, as compared to psoriasis, skin prevents induction of innate immune response genes. *J Immunol*. 2003;171:3262-9.
16. Batista DI, Perez L, Orfali RL, et al. Profile of skin barrier proteins(filaggrin, claudins 1 and 4) and Th1/Th2/Th17 cytokines in adults with atopic dermatitis. *J Eur Acad Dermatol Venereol*. 2015;29:1091-5.

World Clin Dermatol. 2018;4(1):26-36.

Diagnosis and Clinical Features

[1],*Zubin K Mandlewala MBBS DDV, [2]Rashmi Sarkar MD MNAMS

[1]Reflectionz Clinic, Mumbai, Maharashtra, India
[2]Department of Dermatology, Maulana Azad Medical College and
Lok Nayak Hospital, New Delhi, India

ABSTRACT

Atopic dermatitis (AD) is a chronic inflammatory skin disorder characterized primarily by an intense and recurring pruritus that can adversely affect one's quality of life. A complex interplay of various mechanisms, such as genetic, immune, structural, infectious, and environmental, are thought to increasingly contribute to the causation of typical lesions in susceptible individuals. The "itch that rashes" develops in any age group with classical sites of predilection. Although assessment of an atopic by means of an allergen-based skin prick test, skin biopsy, or evaluation of serum immunoglobulin E can be routinely done, such modalities are rarely asked for as the characteristic clinical features itself substantiate the diagnosis of AD. Optimal management of AD requires a multipronged approach aimed at protecting the skin barrier and addressing the symptoms along with the complex immunopathogenetic mechanisms of the disease. Atopic dermatitis in itself can prove to be a psychosocial burden on the patient and family members alike.

INTRODUCTION

Atopic dermatitis (AD, also known as atopic eczema) is a common chronic pruritic inflammatory skin disorder that is more likely to present in infancy (early onset) or childhood, but can also occur in adults (late onset). Atopy is defined as an inherited tendency to produce immunoglobulin E (IgE) antibodies in response to minute amounts of common environmental proteins such as pollen, house dust mites, and food allergens.[1] The disorder exhibits periods of exacerbation and remission. Genetic (e.g., filaggrin gene mutation), immune (e.g., Th2 differentiation of naive CD4+ T cells), and environmental factors (e.g., hygiene hypothesis) interact

---

*Corresponding author
Email: drzman03@gmail.com

in a complex fashion to contribute to disease expression. Currently, it is widely accepted that a defective skin epidermal barrier results in increased transepidermal water loss as well as increased colonization and penetration by microorganisms and allergens, evoking inflammatory responses.[2] The most frequent symptom is pruritus, which induces an intense desire to scratch and thereby development of the classical lesions at age group-specific body areas. This "itch-scratch" cycle can severely hamper one's quality of life; as such symptoms are known to follow a chronic or chronically relapsing course. Along with the social stigma attached therein, AD also causes sleep disturbances that may result in missed days at work or school.

CLINICAL FEATURES

A list of characteristic features was proposed by Hanifin and Rajka in 1980 to establish the diagnosis of atopic dermatitis (Table 1). Atopic dermatitis is often the initial/primary occurrence in the "atopic march" (the sequential development of allergic disease manifestations during early childhood), which further leads to asthma and/or allergic rhinitis in the majority of afflicted patients.[3] Characteristically, an early onset of pruritic lesions localized at typical sites (e.g., face and extensors in infants and flexures of elbows, knees, wrist, and ankles in children and adults) or a strong family history is usually sufficient in

Table 1: Diagnostic features of atopic dermatitis

Major features (3 of 4 present)

1. Pruritus
2. Typical morphology and distribution of skin lesions
3. Chronic or chronically relapsing dermatitis
4. Personal or family history of atopy

Minor features (3 of 23 present)

1. Xerosis
2. Ichthyosis/palmar hyperlinearity/keratosis pilaris
3. Immediate (type I) skin hypersensitivity
4. Elevated serum IgE
5. Early age of onset
6. Tendency towards cutaneous infections/impaired cell-mediated immunity
7. Tendency towards nonspecific hand or foot dermatitis
8. Nipple eczema
9. Cheilitis
10. Recurrent conjunctivitis
11. Dennie-Morgan infraorbital fold
12. Keratoconus
13. Anterior subcapsular cataract
14. Orbital darkening
15. Facial pallor/erythema
16. Pityriasis alba
17. Anterior neck folds
18. Pruritus when sweating
19. Intolerance to wool and lipid solvents
20. Perifollicular accentuation
21. Food intolerance
22. Course influenced by environmental/emotional factors
23. White dermographism/delayed blanch

corroborating a diagnosis of AD. Xerosis occurs due to low water content and an excessive water loss through the epidermis. There are many associated features of AD, commonly referred to as "stigmata." One such associated feature is known as "white dermographism", wherein there is an increased cholinergic response to scratch resulting in hives at the affected site.[1] Another important feature is palmoplantar hyperlinearity (Figure 1), which may be associated with ichthyosis vulgaris and filaggrin mutations. Due mention must be given to a feature known as the Dennie-Morgan fold, which is a double fold of skin underneath the inferior eyelid starting from the inner canthus which is pronounced in times of increased disease activity (Figure 2).[1] The eye surroundings may be darkened (postinflammatory hyperpigmentation) due to repeated inflammatory

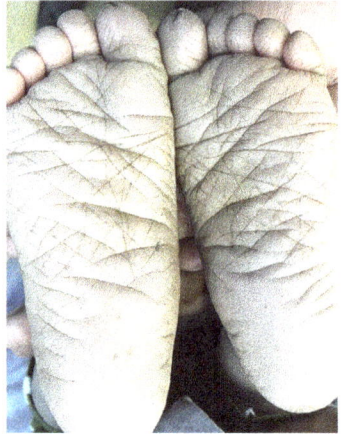

Figure 1: Infantile atopic dermatitis. Plantar hyperlinearity.

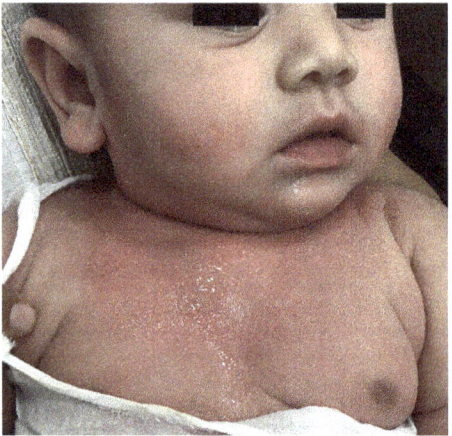

Figure 2: Infantile atopic dermatitis. Dennie-Morgan fold below lower lids. Acute, oozing lesions on a background of erythema.

exacerbations.[1] Upon meticulous examination, some patients may have an associated feature known as Hertoge's sign, which refers to the thinning or absence of the lateral portion of the eyebrows. Atopic dermatitis can be classified into three forms—infantile, childhood, and adulthood. The infantile form usually presents in the first 2–12 months of life. Lesions are intensely pruritic and present as erythematous papules and plaques, surmounted by vesicles and oozing leading to serous crusting (Figure 3). Areas commonly involved are the scalp, cheeks, extensor surfaces of extremities, and the trunk. Lesions of AD usually spare the diaper area. The childhood form is commonly seen in patients between 2 and 12 years of age. It resembles the infantile form early on, but later on evolves into features seen in the adulthood form. The classical sites of involvement are the antecubital and popliteal fossae. In general, lesions are less exudative and patients may present with numerous excoriations, papules, and nodules (Figure 4). Lesions have a gradual shift towards lichenification (Figures 5 and 6). The adulthood form is characterized by subacute to chronic eczematous lesions favoring the flexures, although acute flares of atopic eczema are not uncommon (Figure 7). Lichenification of the neck, wrists, ankles, popliteal fossae, or antecubital fossae is characteristic of chronic atopic dermatitis (Figure 8). It is observed as thickened, leathery, hyperpigmented plaques of skin with a deepening of normal skin creases.[4] The eyelids, retroauricular region, neck, and chest may also be involved. Adult atopics may even present with chronic hand dermatitis. Adults who have progressed in continuum from childhood AD

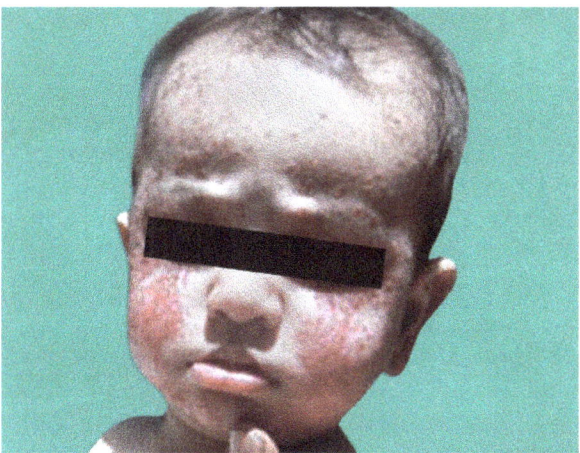

Figure 3: Infantile atopic dermatitis. Erythematous pruritic papules and plaques notably on the cheeks, some of which have led to serous crusting. *Reproduced with permission from:* Zaidi Z, Walton S. A Manual of Dermatology. New Delhi: Jaypee Brothers Medical Publishers Pvt. Ltd; 2015. pp. 216-54.

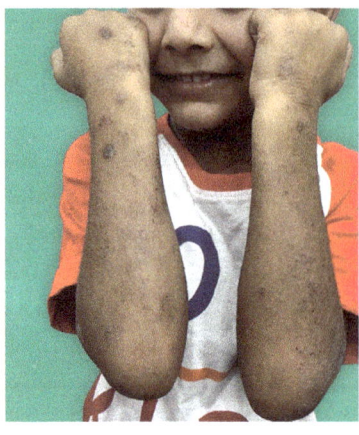

Figure 4: Childhood atopic dermatitis. Multiple crusted excoriation marks. Few, chronic eczematized nummular plaques over hands and forearms.

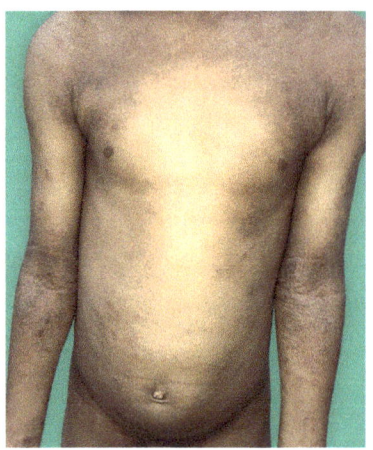

Figure 5: Childhood atopic dermatitis. Hyperpigmented, xerotic, lichenified antecubital fossae and axillary folds.

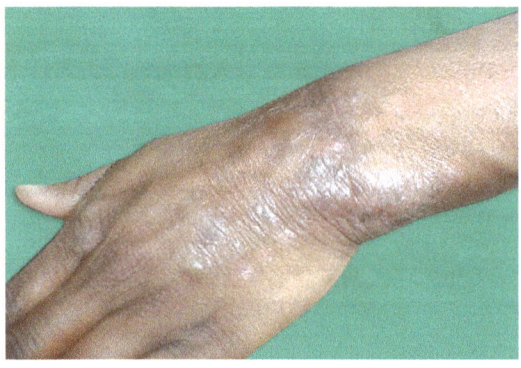

Figure 6: Childhood atopic dermatitis. Chronic atopic eczema leading to hyperpigmented, lichenified skin on the wrist and dorsum of hand. *Reproduced with permission from:* Zaidi Z, Walton S. A Manual of Dermatology. New Delhi: Jaypee Brothers Medical Publishers Pvt. Ltd; 2015. pp. 216-54.

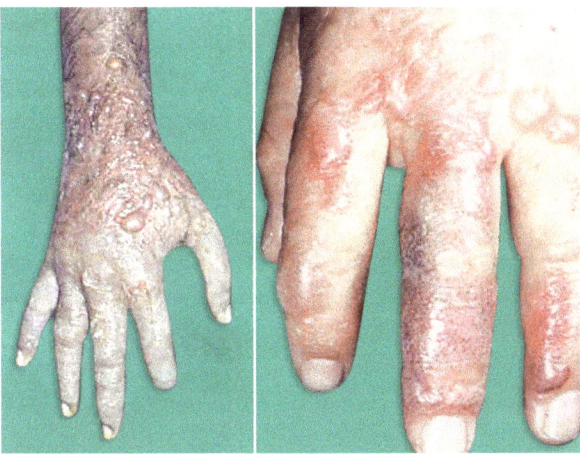

Figure 7: Adult atopic dermatitis. Acute atopic eczema: erythema, vesicles and bullae seen over the forearms and hands. *Reproduced with permission from:* Zaidi Z, Walton S. A Manual of Dermatology. New Delhi: Jaypee Brothers Medical Publishers Pvt. Ltd; 2015. pp. 216-54.

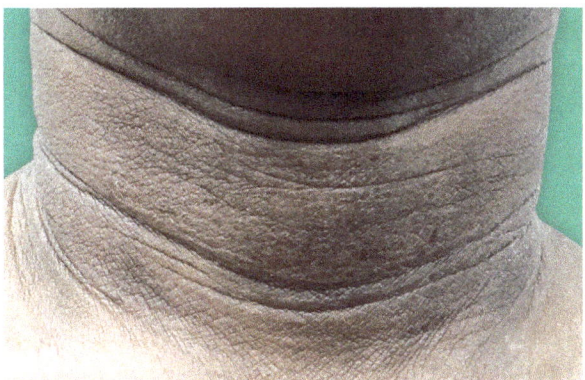

Figure 8: Adult atopic dermatitis. Hyperpigmented, xerotic, lichenified anterior neck folds.

are more at a risk of developing erythrodermic AD. Lesions tend to become more xerotic and less lichenified in senility.

COMPLICATIONS

The skin of atopics is highly prone to secondary infections, the most common of which is colonization with *Staphylococcus aureus* or less commonly with *Streptococcus pyogenes*. The result of such colonization is impetiginization of existing lesions and thereby worsening of disease activity. Sometimes, patients of AD can develop a secondary herpes simplex infection leading to widespread development of pruritic and painful umbilicated papulovesicular eruptions, known as eczema herpeticum or Kaposi's varicelliform eruption. These may develop into pustular or hemorrhagic lesions that may evolve further into painful and confluent erosions with a punched-out appearance. Lesions may occur at any site, but are usually seen on the head, neck, and trunk. The patient invariably is febrile with evidence of lymphadenopathy. Complications of Kaposi's varicelliform eruption include secondary bacterial infection, herpetic keratoconjunctivitis, and meningoencephalitis. A new variant of Kaposi's varicelliform eruption [eczema coxsackium (EC)], attributable to coxsackievirus A6 (CSVA6), is being increasingly recognized. Eczema coxsackium is related to the well-described hand, foot, and mouth disease (HFMD), which is most often caused by CSVA16. Over half of CSVA6-related HFMD manifests as EC.[5] Eczema coxsackium manifests as eczema herpeticum-like lesions with a predilection for hemorrhagic vesicles within dermatitic skin. Patients of AD are also predisposed to develop widespread molluscum contagiosum. Apart from infections, atopics can develop various ocular abnormalities such as keratoconjunctivitis, blepharitis, subcapsular cataract (posterior > anterior in AD), keratoconus, and very rarely, retinal detachment. Reports of systemic and cutaneous lymphomas developing in a few patients of AD have surfaced and need to be further investigated. One of the most important complications of AD that is often overlooked is the psychosocial effect(s). In children the pruritus at times becomes so severe that it cause routine sleep disturbance and thus results in missed days at school. Even at school, the child may feel isolated, as teachers fear the disorder may be communicable. Other school children may also start teasing the atopic child affecting his/her self-esteem. As a consequence of such physical and mental agony, the child is likely to develop many behavioral problems. At times, growth delay has also been observed in such children. Quite understandably, as the child is disturbed, the parents become emotionally distressed. Adult atopics also deal relatively with the same psychosocial aspects, causing numerous days missed at work. Irritability, anxiety, and depression are all complications of AD and thus can negatively hamper one's quality of life.

DIFFERENTIAL DIAGNOSIS

Usually, the distribution and morphology of lesions along with a detailed history provided by the patient are sufficient in formulating a diagnosis of AD. Yet, one must keep in mind a few potential differentials such as scabies, seborrheic dermatitis, and psoriasis (Table 2), in not so evident cases. Infantile scabies is usually distinguished by the presence of burrows, small-crusted papules, or vesiculopustular lesions acrally and a predominantly nocturnal itch. Many a times,

Table 2: Differential diagnosis of atopic dermatitis	
Infections	• Scabies • Dermatophytosis • Impetigo • HIV-associated dermatoses
Inflammatory dermatoses	• Psoriasis • Seborrheic dermatitis • Contact dermatitis • Lichen simplex chronicus • Nummular dermatitis
Immunodeficiencies	• Wiskott-Aldrich syndrome • Hyper-IgE syndrome • Severe combined immunodeficiency syndrome • Ataxia telangiectasia
Autoimmune	• Pemphigus foliaceus • Dermatitis herpetiformis • Dermatomyositis • Lupus erythematosus
Congenital	• Netherton's syndrome
Metabolic	• Acrodermatitis enteropathica (zinc deficiency) • Phenylketonuria • Pyridoxine (vitamin B6) • Pellagra (niacin deficiency)
Malignancies	• Cutaneous T-cell lymphoma • Langerhans cell histiocytosis
Other	• Chronic actinic dermatitis • Photoallergic contact dermatitis

HIV, human immunodeficiency virus; IgE, immunoglobulin E.

a family member may be suffering concurrently from the same scabetic infestation, which is usually not the case in AD. Infantile seborrheic dermatitis (SD) can accompany AD or even precede it. Yellowish adherent scale-crusts are likely to be seen on the scalp in infantile seborrheic dermatitis (Figure 9). Seborrheic dermatitis is usually distinguished by a lack of excoriations and sleep impairment. Another important distinguishing point is that lesions of SD usually resolve by two years of age. Seborrheic dermatitis in adolescents and adults characteristically involves the scalp as well as alar and mesolabial folds. Nail involvement and lesion in diaper area help differentiate infantile psoriasis from AD. Adult psoriatics will more commonly present with involvement of the extensor joints (e.g., elbows and knees), palms and soles, nails, lower back, and/or scalp. Psoriatic plaques are indurated, sharply circumscribed, and are surmounted with silvery-white adherent scales that are relatively absent in adult AD. Histopathology can with certainty aid in differentiating psoriasis from AD.

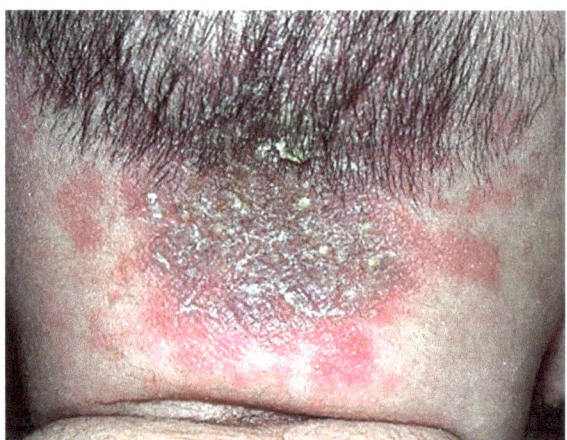

Figure 9: Infantile seborrheic dermatitis. Characteristic yellow adherent greasy scaling, which must be differentiated from infantile atopic dermatitis. *Reproduced with permission from:* Zaidi Z, Walton S. A Manual of Dermatology. New Delhi: Jaypee Brothers Medical Publishers Pvt. Ltd; 2015. pp. 216-54.

DIAGNOSIS

Atopic dermatitis is primarily a clinical diagnosis, as pathognomic biomarkers for AD are yet to be identified. Clinically, the Scoring Atopic Dermatitis (SCORAD) index is the most commonly used clinical tool to assess the extent and severity of atopic eczema (Table 3). Other validated scoring systems include EASI (Eczema Area Scoring Index) and POEM (Patient-Oriented Eczema Measure). In terms of laboratory assessment, estimation of total and specific IgE usually serves only to confirm the atopic nature of the individual. Similarly, a positive skin prick test (SPT) may indicate sensitization to a particular allergen but it does not prove clinical hypersensitivity or causation. For children with moderate to severe AD where a plausible and/or near certain food allergy exists, it is prudent to check for sensitivity to eggs, milk, peanuts, soy, wheat, fish, and tree nuts (walnut, cashew, pecan) by using skin prick tests or RAST (Radio Allergo Sorbent Test).[6,7] Likewise, exposure to aeroallergens such as house dust mites, animal dander, pollen, and moulds can exacerbate AD in some patients. Here again, if sensitization is established by means of an SPT along with a highly suggestive history leading to exacerbation of AD, then specific avoidance measures should be considered. Withdrawal of exposure from the aeroallergen would, in all likelihood, improve the symptoms of AD. Patch testing is a procedure that can be utilized when an atopic concurrently develops contact dermatitis, but seldom should it be used as a primary investigative technique in AD. A skin biopsy is not of diagnostic use as all forms of dermatitis, regardless of cause, show relatively the

Table 3: Scoring Atopic Dermatitis index

Area

Score of each affected area is added up and thus total area is "**A**"
Maximum = 100%)

- Head and neck: 9%
- Upper limbs: 9% each
- Lower limbs: 18% each
- Anterior trunk: 18%
- Back: 18%
- Genitals: 1%

Intensity

Intensity of each of the following signs is assessed as none (0), mild (1), moderate (2) or severe (3). Intensity scores are added up to give "**B**"
Maximum = 18)

- Erythema
- Edema
- Oozing/crusting
- Excoriations
- Lichenification
- Dryness (assessed in an area devoid of inflammation)

Subjective symptoms

Each symptom is scored by the patient or relative using a visual analog scale where (0) is no itch (or no sleeplessness) and (10) is the worst imaginable itch (or sleeplessness). These scores are added to give "**C**"
Maximum = 20)

- Pruritus
- Sleeplessness

Total score: The SCORAD for an individual is A/5 + 7B/2 + C

same histological features. On biopsy, an acute atopic will demonstrate spongiosis, perivascular lymphocytic infiltration, and parakeratosis; whereas a chronic atopic will demonstrate features of hyperkeratosis, acanthosis, and very few lymphocytic infiltrates. Where bacterial colonization is suspected, a swab of infected skin may help with the isolation of a specific organism (e.g., *Staphylococcus* > *Streptococcus*). Thereafter, it can be subjected to antibiotic sensitivity for a better treatment outcome. Similarly, a swab for viral polymerase chain reaction may help identify superinfection with herpes simplex virus, which can be essential in substantiating a diagnosis of eczema herpeticum.

CONCLUSION

Atopic dermatitis is a common chronic skin disorder in which one symptom, pruritus, with all its might, is enough to cause many physical and psychosocial detrimental effects to children and adults alike. Where certain plausible triggers such as food or aeroallergens are implicated, testing for these may certainly aid in reduction of further disease progression. It is also imperative to manage atopic skin with due respect to the etiological factors responsible for the initiation/progression of the disorder. As a defective skin barrier is centrally paramount in all cases, appropriate and regular skin care is highly advised to prevent any undue complications therein.

Editor's Comment

Recognition of minor features of atopic dermatitis is important in identifying an individual with an "atopic diathesis". This would help in preventing a more severe form of disease if the right general measures are followed. Recognition of atypical features, and regional differences in clinical features pertinent to an area is important.

Rashmi Sarkar

REFERENCES

1. Thomsen SF. Atopic dermatitis: Natural history, diagnosis, and treatment. *ISRN Allergy.* 2014;2014:354250.
2. Boguniewicz M, Leung DY. Atopic dermatitis: A disease of altered skin barrier and immune dysregulation. *Immunol Rev.* 2011;242(1):233-46.
3. Spergel JM, Paller AS. Atopic dermatitis and the atopic march. *J Allergy Clin Immunol.* 2003;112:S128-39.
4. Glazenburg EJ, Mulder PG, Oranje AP. A statistical model to predict the reduction of lichenification in atopic dermatitis. *Acta Derm Venereol.* 2015;95(3):294-7.
5. Mathes EF, Oza V, Frieden IJ, et al. "Eczema coxsackium" and unusual cutaneous findings in an enterovirus outbreak. *Pediatrics.* 2013;132:e149-57.
6. Jones SM, Burks W. Atopic dermatitis and food hypersensitivity. In: Pediatric allergy: Principles and practice. St. Louis, Inc.: Mosby; 2003. pp. 538-45.
7. Krakowski AC, Eichenfield LF, Dohil MA. Management of atopic dermatitis in the pediatric population. *Pediatrics.* 2008;122:812-24.

World Clin Dermatol. 2018;4(1):37-45.

Severity Scoring in Atopic Dermatitis

Pallavi Ailawadi MD DNB

Department of Dermatology and STD
Maulana Azad Medical College and Associate Hospitals, New Delhi, India

ABSTRACT

Atopic dermatitis (AD) is a common chronic inflammatory skin disease and is an important health problem worldwide, especially in children. Symptoms like pruritus and skin lesions can be severe and intractable, leading to emotional distress, sleep loss, and social stigma. These depend on the severity of the disease, measurement of which is of great significance, both for research purposes and routine clinical practice. Multiple outcome measures and tools have been used to grade the severity of AD. This article reviews the common scoring methods used for comprehensive assessment of disease severity in AD.

INTRODUCTION

Atopic dermatitis (AD) is a common chronic inflammatory skin disease which is an important health problem worldwide. The incidence of AD appears to be increasing globally and a similar trend has been observed in India. Atopic dermatitis is more frequent among children with most of the patients developing the disease in infancy, as seen in up to 60% of cases and onset before 5 years of age is seen in up to 85%.[1] The prevalence and severity of the disease usually decreases with age.

Atopic dermatitis encompasses an array of features. Pruritus is considered to be an essential component. Cutaneous lesions of AD can be classified as acute, subacute, and chronic. Acute AD is characterized by pruritic papules and papulovesicles with serous exudates on a background of erythema. Subacute eczema is characterized by either grouped or scattered scaly, erythematous papules, or plaques over an erythematous skin. Chronic AD includes thickening of the skin

---

Email: apallavi99@gmail.com

with lichenification, secondary to scratching and rubbing. The distribution and extent of the lesions varies with severity of the disease.

Chronicity is characteristic of AD and this affects patients' physical and psychosocial wellbeing and severe disease can adversely affect social and personal relationships. The symptoms of atopic dermatitis, notably pruritus, can be intractable and lead to significant emotional distress and sleep loss. Further, the clinical signs of erythematous oozy or dark lichenified lesions on visible body parts also add to the stigma felt by the patients.

DISEASE SEVERITY MEASUREMENT

The measurement of severity of disease and its impact on the patient's lives is of great significance, both in the clinical trial setting and for monitoring response to therapy in routine clinical practice. These are also important in studying the impact of disease on the patients as well as their quality of life, economic aspects of treatment, and plays a role in allocation of resources in healthcare. Therefore, assessing the severity of AD in objective and reproducible manner is extremely important. Clinically, the severity of the disease can be assessed by measuring the extent of the disease (body surface area involvement) as well by evaluating the severity of the lesions and various clinical signs. In addition to these objective measurements, subjective component of the disease, the symptoms as perceived by the patient can also be assessed to evaluate the overall impact of the disease on the patient. There is no gold standard measure of AD severity, and all these components should be taken into account. The physical features of disease as well as subjective indicators are given higher significance compared to extent of the disease. Apart from these clinical parameters, there is no accepted laboratory test or marker of disease activity. Multiple outcome measures and tools have been used to grade the severity of AD in clinical practice as well as trials. In clinical trials, detailed tools which assess all parameters are preferred, whereas for routine clinical use, simpler indices are more useful.

TOOLS FOR MEASUREMENT OF DISEASE SEVERITY

Various scales have been developed overtime for measurement of AD severity. The common ones include Severity Scoring of Atopic Dermatitis (SCORAD) index, Eczema Area and Severity Index (EASI), Investigators' Global Assessment (IGA), Patient-Oriented Eczema Measurement (POEM), Three Item Severity Score (TIS), and Six Area, Six Sign Atopic Dermatitis (SASSAD). Apart from these disease specific instruments, some AD nonspecific scales like Visual Analogue Scale (VAS), Pruritus Numerical-Rating Scale (PNRS), and Pruritus Categorical Response Scale (PCRS) have also been used.

As per a systematic review on recent trends in disease severity tools used in randomized control trials (RCTs) on patients with AD (between July, 2010 and July, 2015), 62 disease severity scales were used in the 135 reviewed RCTs. The most frequently used disease severity scale was the SCORAD index, which was used in 79 (59%) studies, while the second most common instrument was the VAS for pruritus (n = 30). These were closely followed by the IGA tool (n = 29) and the EASI (n = 28). Forty-five of the identified disease severity scales were used in only one study.[2]

The number of scales used has drastically risen overtime, as can be seen from a review of 382 RCTs on AD treatment published between 1985 and July, 2010 in which only 20 disease severity scales were identified. In this review also, SCORAD was the most frequently used scale; it was used in 113 out of 382 RCTs (30%). The next most frequent scale was the EASI which was used in 63 (16%) RCTs, followed by the IGA that was used in 48 (13%) studies and SASSAD used in 18 (5%) RCTs. These four scales were used in the majority of RCTs—242 out of 382 (63%), whereas, the remaining 14 scales were used in 57 out of 382 RCTs (15%).[3]

During the process of scale development it undergoes rigorous testing and evaluation of the following statistical properties: validity (construct, content, convergent, and concurrent), inter-and intra-rater reliability, internal consistency reliability, responsiveness to change, and minimal clinically important difference. Validity is defined as the extent to which the scores from a measure represent the variable they are intended to, i.e., suitability or meaningfulness of the measurement and if the instrument describes accurately the construct it is attempting to measure. Reliability refers to the consistency of a measure and repeatability of the scoring system in different circumstances. As per the findings of a systematic review on measurement properties of outcome measurements for clinical signs of AD statistically the EASI and SCORAD are the best instruments to assess the clinical signs of AD with respect to the validity and reliability.[4]

The important scales have been explained in brief to allow the readers to have a basic understanding of these tools and basic method of measurement.

Severity Scoring of Atopic Dermatitis

This index was developed in 1993 by the European Task Force on atopic dermatitis.[5] It is a comprehensive score that assesses both objective and subjective components of the disease severity. The SCORAD index uses the rule of nines to measure body surface area (BSA) involvement to assess disease extent and evaluate five clinical characteristics to determine disease severity: (i) erythema, (ii) edema/papulation, (iii) oozing/crusts, (iv) excoriation, and (5) lichenification; on a scale of 0–3, each measured at a single representative body site. SCORAD also assesses subjective symptoms of pruritus and sleep loss with VAS on the scale of 0–10. The total

SCORAD score is calculated as: BSA/5 + 7 (the sum of intensity scores)/2 + the subjective symptom score, to give a maximum possible score of 103. Although, it is a combined score of objective and subjective components, the scores can be separated and used individually. It is the most widely used disease severity scale in AD and of all the scales it is also the most widely validated disease-severity instrument.[2,4] SCORAD has been found to be valid and reliable, and it has shown excellent agreement with global assessments of disease severity.[3-7] However, some studies have shown interobserver variation in scoring lichenification and extent of disease.[5,6]

The SCORAD index can be calculated by filling in the details of the patient on a premade proforma as well as through multiple software available online (http://www.fondation-dermatite-atopique.org/en/healthcare-professionals-space/scorad). With adequate training, assessment of the score can be made within a short time i.e., less than 10 minutes.[8] Recently, a self-assessed patient-oriented version of SCORAD was created by the European Task Force on atopic dermatitis, validated in 2011 (PO-SCORAD).[9] It is completed by the patients themselves, either through a printed proforma or a computer software (http://www.fondation-dermatite-atopique.org/en/healthcare-professionals-space/po-scorad). The PO-SCORAD evaluates the condition of AD over the last 3 days. Although, a multicenter study has proven that SCORAD completed by doctors and the PO-SCORAD completed by patients are indeed correlated, some clinical signs were found to be difficult for self-assessment, like disease extent, lichenification, and edema/swelling of the skin.[9]

Eczema Area and Severity Index

The eczema area and severity index (EASI) score was developed in 1998 as a tool for assessing severity of AD and monitoring response to treatment.[10] EASI, as a disease severity measurement tool, evaluates two dimensions of AD—disease extent and clinical signs. It assesses extent of disease at four body sites and measures four clinical signs: (i) erythema, (ii) induration/papulation, (iii) excoriation, and (iv) lichenification each on a scale of 0–3. Disease extent is also assessed in each of the four regions on a scale of 0–6. The sum of the scores for each body region gives the EASI total maximum score of 72. EASI is an objective score and does not assess subjective symptoms. It is among the four most commonly used disease severity scales in AD trials.[2,3] EASI has been found to have excellent validity, internal consistency, and sensitivity to change.[11] While EASI is a valid and reliable instrument, most interobserver variability lies in the dimension of induration/population.[10,11] A self-assessed version of the EASI (SA-EASI) has been proposed for parents or caregivers of patients under 12 years of age as well as patients older than 12 years.[12] It provides the caregivers the means to report the severity of their child's skin disease, objectively. It shows reasonable correlation between parental and physician-assessed scores but poor agreement between individual components of the scale.[12,13]

Investigators' Global Assessment

Investigators' Global Assessment is a tool for global assessment of the severity of AD on an ordinal scale. It evaluates clinical characteristics of (i) erythema, (ii) infiltration, (iii) papulation, (iv) oozing, and (v) crusting for overall severity assessment of the disease. It consists of a 6-point severity scale, ranging from clear to very severe disease.[14]

It is the second most commonly used disease severity scale in RCTs on AD as per a recent systematic review.[2] Apart from studies, ease of its use makes in a commonly used instrument in routine clinical practice to grade the severity of AD as well as monitor response to therapy. Furthermore, by virtue of being an easy-to-comprehend scale, it provides a readily understandable measure of overall severity, both for the patient and the physician.

Although, IGA has not been validated as an outcome measure it has been used to validate other outcome scales as one gold standard.[11] IGA appears to correlate well with the EASI and is considered an instrument with reasonable face validity. The demerits of this scale include lack of responsiveness and discrimination for disease severity and lack of subjective symptoms.

Patient-Oriented Eczema Measure

The POEM is a simple and readily understandable tool for monitoring disease severity in patients with AD which was developed to help address the imbalance between physician and patient-based outcome measures in AD. It incorporates seven symptoms: itching, sleep disturbance, bleeding, weeping, cracking, flaking, and dryness of the skin using a simple 5-point scale of frequency of occurrence during the previous week.[15] The POEM is scored by patients (or parents) over a 1-week period, with a maximum possible score of 28. Due to the simplicity of use it can be used in routine clinical practice as well as in clinical trials. The questionnaires and scoring sheets are available free on the United Kingdom Centre for Evidence Based Dermatology website (http://www.nottingham.ac.uk/scs/divisions/evidencebaseddermatology/resources/patientorientedeczemameasure.aspx) and translations are available on the Patient-Reported Outcome and Quality of Life Instruments Database (http://www.proqolid.org). It has demonstrated good validity and repeatability in adults and children ranging from 1 year of age, upwards. Further research is needed to provide information on the clinical meaning of individual scores, both for entry into clinical trials and outcome analysis.

Other Scales

Multiple scales have been developed to assess the severity of AD. Going into the details of all indices would be beyond the realms of this article. However, apart from the above mentioned indices, two more deserve a brief mention.

The SASSAD index is a widely used score comprising an assessment of six clinical signs: erythema, exudation, excoriation, dryness, cracking, and lichenification. It is measured at six defined body sites including arms, hands, legs, feet, head and neck, and trunk, each on a scale of 0–3; 0 (absent), 1 (mild), 2 (moderate), or 3 (severe) giving a maximum score of 108.[16] The measurement of clinical signs at six body sites rather than a single representative site, provides an indirect estimate of disease extent without the need for precise measurement of BSA involvement. It has been found to be a valid and reliable index.[17]

The TIS score is a rough but simple and reliable scoring tool for AD which involves the scoring of erythema, edema, and excoriations on a scale from 0 to 3, at one representative lesion. The range of the TIS score lies between 0 and 9. It corresponds well with the objective of SCORAD.[18] It is particularly suitable in routine clinical use, screening purposes in clinical trials, and is excellent for epidemiological studies.

WHICH SCALE TO USE?

Different scoring systems have been developed to determine the severity of AD and all of them have their own strengths and weaknesses. The choice of the scale depends on the purpose of its use. In clinical trials, detailed tools which provide comprehensive assessment of the disease are preferred, whereas for routine clinical use, simpler indices are more useful.

Currently, the three most adequately validated and tested outcome measures for AD are the SCORAD index, EASI, and POEM.[2-4,7] While the objectives of SCORAD and EASI indicate physician evaluated assessment of the disease, POEM is fully patient-derived and patient-assessed. All three of them provide complementary information on AD severity.[2-4,7]

Recently, consensus-based sets of core outcome domains for AD for use in controlled trials and clinical record keeping have been developed. The Harmonizing Outcomes Measures for Eczema (HOME) initiative has identified four core outcomes which are recommended for inclusion in all future AD trials in order to enhance clinical interpretability and to enable meta-analyses across different studies: (i) patient symptoms, (ii) physician-assessed clinical signs, (iii) quality of life, and (iv) measurement for long-term control of flares.[19]

The core outcome measure for the clinical signs domain should include erythema, excoriation, edema/population, and lichenification as a minimum to achieve content validity. Both the intensity and extent of each clinical sign in the core set should be measured. It has been agreed that EASI scale should be the core outcome measure instrument for clinician reported signs in AD, at HOME III in San Diego. The EASI was favored over objective SCORAD because (i) no requirement to identify a representative site; (ii) measures only the four essential signs; (iii) more importance is given to extent; and (iv) distinguishing between body areas may be important in future research.[19]

As per the most recent consensus statement from the HOME IV meeting held in April 2015, the POEM scale was voted as adequate for measuring the patient reported symptoms of AD in clinical trials and therefore, is to be recommended for inclusion in the core outcome set. The symptoms of itch, sleep loss, dryness, redness/inflamed skin, and irritated skin are all essential for measuring AD.[20]

Although, a global assessment has not been recommended as a core outcome by the HOME group, the US FDA recommends that an IGA serve as the primary end point for trials supporting new drug applications for AD.

OTHER MEASURES OF DISEASE SEVERITY

Apart from the above mentioned scales, several other methods can be used to assess the severity of the disease. These include several objective criteria as well as biological parameters. Objective measures include skin hydration, skin pH, and transepidermal water loss.[21-23] The serum levels of several biomarkers have been recently found to correlate with the severity of the disease and measurement of the same would give a fair idea of the activity of the disease. They can be utilized to monitor disease activity and clinical response to an intervention or as a surrogate endpoint in clinical trials. These markers, including serum eosinophil cationic protein, soluble E-selectin, CD30, interleukin (IL)-12, IL-16, IL-18, IL-31, and thymus and activation-regulated chemokine and macrophage-derived chemokine, have demonstrated correlation with AD disease severity and may provide additional information on disease activity.[24] However, due to lack of reliable sensitivity or specificity for AD, they are not used routinely as they cannot support diagnosis or monitoring of the disease.

CONCLUSION

During the treatment of a chronic disease with a relapsing remitting course like AD, clinical scoring systems add to the armamentarium of the physician as they are useful tools in grading both severity of the disease and monitoring response to treatment, both in routine clinical practice as well as clinical trials. Despite a plethora of tools available, a single best scoring system for all purposes is not available. The SCORAD, EASI, and POEM are the best available systems.

Further research is required to establish the role of serum biomarkers and other biological parameters in determining the severity of AD. It is a long way to go to develop that one ideal scoring system for all purposes.

Editor's Comment

The measurement of severity of disease and its impact on the patient's lives is of great significance, both in the clinical trial setting and for monitoring response to therapy in routine clinical practice. These are also important in studying the impact of disease on the patients, as well as their quality of life. Economic aspects of treatment play a role in allocation of resources in healthcare. Scoring Atopic Dermatitis (SCORAD), Eczema Area and Severity Index (EASI), and Visual Analogue Scale (VAS) for pruritus remain important scales for subjectively scoring pruritus.

Rashmi Sarkar

REFERENCES

1. Rajka G. Essential aspects of atopic dermatitis. Berlin: Springer Verlag; 1989. p. 1.
2. Hill MK, Pishkenari AZ, Braunberger TL, et al. Recent trends in disease severity and quality of life instruments for patients with atopic dermatitis: A systematic review. *J Am Acad Dermatol*. 2016;7:906-17.
3. Rehal B, Armstrong AW. Health outcome measures in atopic dermatitis: A systematic review of trends in disease severity and quality-of-life instruments 1985-2010. *PLoS One*. 2011;6:e17520.
4. Schmitt J, Langan S, Deckert S, et al. Assessment of clinical signs of atopic dermatitis: A systematic review and recommendation. *J Allergy Clin Immunol*. 2013;132:1337-47.
5. Kunz B, Oranje AP, Labrèze L, et al. Clinical validation and guidelines for the SCORAD index: Consensus report of the European Task Force on atopic dermatitis. *Dermatology*. 1997;195:10-9.
6. Charman C, Williams H. Outcome measures of disease severity in atopic eczema. *Arch Dermatol*. 2000;136:763-9.
7. Schmitt J, Langan S, Williams HC. What are the best outcome measurements for atopic eczema? A systematic review. *J Allergy Clin Immunol*. 2007;120:1389-98.
8. Oranje AP, Stalder JF, Taïeb A, et al. Scoring of atopic dermatitis by SCORAD using a training atlas by investigators from different disciplines. *Pediatr Allergy Immunol*. 1997;8:28-34.
9. Stalder JF, Barbarot S, Wollenberg A, et al. Patient-Oriented SCORAD (PO-SCORAD): A new self-assessment scale in atopic dermatitis validated in Europe. *Allergy*. 2011;66:1114-21.
10. Hanifin JM, Thurston M, Omoto M, et al. The eczema area and severity index (EASI): assessment of reliability in atopic dermatitis. EASI Evaluator Group. *Exp Dermatol*. 2001;10:11-8.
11. Barbier N, Paul C, Luger T, et al. Validation of the Eczema Area and Severity Index for atopic dermatitis in a cohort of 1550 patients from the pimecrolimus cream 1% randomized controlled clinical trials programme. *Br J Dermatol*. 2004;150:96-102.
12. Housman TS, Patel MJ, Camacho F, et al. Use of the Self-Administered Eczema Area and Severity Index by parent caregivers: results of a validation study. *Br J Dermatol*. 2002;147:1192-8.
13. Van Velsen SG, Knol MJ, Haeck IM, et al. The Self-administered Eczema Area and Severity Index in children with moderate to severe atopic dermatitis: better estimation of AD body surface area than severity. *Pediatr Dermatol*. 2010;27:470-5.

14. Eichenfield LF, Lucky AW, Boguniewicz M, et al. Safety and efficacy of pimecrolimus (ASM 981) cream 1% in the treatment of mild and moderate atopic dermatitis in children and adolescents. *J Am Acad Dermatol.* 2002;46:495-504.
15. Charman CR, Venn AJ, Williams HC. The patient-oriented eczema measure: Development and initial validation of a new tool for measuring atopic eczema severity from the patients' perspective. *Arch Dermatol.* 2004;140:1513-9.
16. Berth-Jones J. Six area, six sign atopic dermatitis (SASSAD) severity score: a simple system for monitoring disease activity in atopic dermatitis. *Br J Dermatol.* 1996;135:25-30.
17. Charman CR, Venn AJ, Williams HC. Reliability testing of the Six Area, Six Sign Atopic Dermatitis severity score. *Br J Dermatol.* 2003;146:1057-60.
18. Wolkerstorfer A, de Waard van der Spek FB, Glazenburg EJ, et al. Scoring the severity of atopic dermatitis: Three item severity score as a rough system for daily practice and as a pre-screening tool for studies. *Acta Derm Venereol.* 1999;79:356-9.
19. JR Chalmers, J Schmitt, C Apfelbacher, et al. Report from the third international consensus meeting to harmonise core outcome measures for atopic eczema/dermatitis clinical trials (HOME). *Br J Dermatol.* 2014;171:1318-25.
20. Chalmers JR, Simpson E, Apfelbacher CJ, et al. Report from the fourth international consensus meeting to harmonize core outcome measures or atopic eczema/dermatitis clinical trials (HOME initiative). *Br J Dermatol.* 2016;175:69-79.
21. Hon KL, Wong KY, Leung TF, et al. Comparison of skin hydration evaluation sites and correlations among skin hydration, transepidermal water loss, SCORAD Index, Nottingham Eczema Severity Score, and quality of life in patients with atopic dermatitis. *Am J Clin Dermatol.* 2008;9:45-50.
22. Holm EA, Wulf HC, Thomassen L, et al. Assessment of atopic eczema: clinical scoring and non-invasive measurements. *Br J Dermatol.* 2007;157:674-80.
23. Holm EA, Wulf HC, Thomassen L, et al. Instrumental assessment of atopic eczema: Validation of trans-epidermal water loss, stratum corneum hydration, erythema, scaling, and edema. *J Am Acad Dermatol.* 2006;55:772-80.
24. Eichenfield LF, Tom WL, Chamlin SL, et al. Guidelines of care for the management of atopic dermatitis: Part 1: Diagnosis and Assessment of Atopic Dermatitis. *J Am Acad Dermatol.* 2014;70:338-51.

World Clin Dermatol. 2018;4(1):46-58.

Investigations in Atopic Eczema

Akanksha Kaushik MD, *Rahul Mahajan MD

Department of Dermatology, Venereology, and Leprology
Postgraduate Institute of Medical Education and Research, Chandigarh, India

ABSTRACT

Atopic dermatitis (AD) is a chronic, relapsing inflammatory disorder of skin, affecting all age groups and a lifetime prevalence approaching 20%. Although the diagnosis is primarily clinical, the disease often deviates from typical clinical patterns, especially in adult-onset AD. Classically, the role of investigations like serum immunoglobulin E and prick test has been indicating the atopic diathesis in the patient, but these are not considered diagnostic. Since disruption of epithelial barrier and subsequent inflammation play a pivotal role in AD, newer investigations focussing on these biomarkers can help to identify trigger factors for flares in AD, as well as determine prognosis and outcome in a patient with AD. The article presents a comprehensive review of the investigation modalities available in AD, including the role of biomarkers.

INTRODUCTION

Atopic dermatitis (AD) is a common, chronic inflammatory disorder of skin, affecting both children and adults worldwide. The disease is characterized by periodic flares requiring medical attention and significantly affects quality of life in the affected patients. The diagnosis of AD is primarily clinical.[1] However, a marker like serum IgE is included as minor criteria in the Hanifin and Rajka clinical criteria and also helps to classify disease as intrinsic or extrinsic, thereby affecting prognosis. Hence investigations in AD can have a role in diagnosis, classification, and prognosis. Investigations are also important in identifying the triggers of AD and in assessing comorbidities. The present review aims to summarize the role of investigations in AD, including patch tests and prick tests. The review also gives an insight into the potential future biomarkers which may have an upcoming role in management of AD patients.

*Corresponding author
Email: drrahulpgi@yahoo.com

DIAGNOSIS

Diagnosis of AD is made clinically, based upon the patient's clinical and family history, as well as clinical examination. A widely used criteria to diagnose AD is that given by Hanifin and Rajka in 1980. This criterion used clinical symptoms of AD, divided into major and minor criteria. Despite their usefulness, there were some shortcomings. The criteria were found to be useful in hospital setting but limitations were seen in population-based studies. Also, the criteria were cumbersome and time-consuming. The criteria were refined by Williams et al. to formulate the United Kingdom Working Party's Diagnostic Criteria and the modifications were found to be validated in both population based studies as well as hospital settings.[2-4] An Indian study reported statistical advantage for Hanifin and Rajka criteria, with better sensitivity for diagnosis of AD, as compared to the UK working party's criteria.[5] In addition, various other clinical criteria have been proposed for the diagnosis of AD. In 1989, Kang and Tian proposed a set of criteria for diagnosis of AD in Chinese patients, which was based upon slight modifications in the Hanifin and Rakja criteria.[6] The Schultz-Larsen criteria consisting of statements and questions, with a certain point value attached to these, were proposed in 1992. The Lillehammer criteria were proposed by Schultz-Larsen, Diepgen, and Svensson in 1994. However, both these criteria are not validated and are not widely used. The International Study of Asthma and Allergies in Childhood (ISAAC) criteria, based on questionnaire method is primarily used in epidemiological studies assessing prevalence of AD. Japanese Dermatology Association criteria gave a set of criteria, based upon features like pruritus, typical morphology, and chronic or chronically relapsing course and were further revised in 2008.[7] In 1998, the Millennium criteria were proposed, in which the presence of allergen-specific IgE was stated to be mandatory for diagnosis of AD.[8] Another set of criteria, the Danish Allergy Research Centre (DARC) criteria were proposed in 2005. The more commonly used criteria for the diagnosis of AD are summarized in table 1.

Table 1: List of Major Diagnostic Criteria Proposed for Atopic Dermatitis

- Hanifin and Rajka criteria, 1980
- Kang and Tian criteria, 1989
- Schultz-Larsen criteria, 1992
- Lillehammer criteria, 1994
- The UK diagnostic criteria, 1994
- International Study of Asthma and Allergies in Childhood questionnaire, 1995
- Japanese Dermatology Association criteria, 1994, 2008
- Millenium diagnostic criteria, 1998
- Danish Allergy Research Centre, 2005

The role of investigations in AD is limited. Laboratory investigations, provocation tests, and skin tests are useful to identify allergens responsible for precipitating AD. Recent research has focused on identifying potential biomarkers for AD, both diagnostic and prognostic.

Serum Immunoglobulin E

The total serum immunoglobulin E (IgE) is found to be elevated in almost 80% patients with AD. Total IgE levels between 6 and 18 months age can predict subsequent clinical AD at 5 years of age. Since IgE values show large variations even among patients with AD, no fixed cutoffs have been defined. The total serum IgE does not correlate with short-term activity but elevated values are good indicators of activity and long-term severity of AD.[7] Broadly, two patterns of AD are seen. First is the intrinsic variant, where allergen-specific IgE is not detected, due to lack of IgE-mediated sensitization. Second variety is the extrinsic type, commonly seen in children, where allergen-specific IgE is detected. There is reported significant correlation between total serum IgE and allergen-specific IgE levels.[9] Kiiski et al. have reported poor long-term outcome in patients with elevated total IgE in AD.[10] In a recent study, significant correlation between AD severity (measured by SCORAD) and serum total IgE levels was found in both childhood and adult AD patients. Specific IgE levels for *Malassezia species* were also found to be elevated in children with AD in the same study.[11] The recent review by Thijs et al. reported weak correlation of serum total IgE levels with severity of AD on follow up.[12]

Banerjee et al. recently observed significant elevation of specific IgE antibodies against Der p 11 allergen in house dust mite allergic patients with AD.[13] Mittermann et al. too observed a significant difference in IgE sensitization profile between severe and moderate AD in adults and proposed a potential role of molecular profiling of sensitization patterns in adult AD patients. Severe AD patients were reported to react to a larger panel of environmental allergens and showed higher IgE-reactivity to skin-associated microorganisms like *Malassezia sympodialis* and *Staphylococcus aureus*.[14]

Some studies have evaluated the role of radio allergo sorbent testing (RAST) in AD. Ohman and Johansson showed specific IgE against various air-borne and food allergens using RAST test in AD.[15] Similar results were reported by Takahashi et al.[16] They further demonstrated greater number of positive RAST reactions in patients with high serum IgE and coexisting asthma/allergic rhinitis. Positive reactions against house dust mite have been reported in many patients. Rudzki and Litewska have reported that frequency of positive RAST for food allergens decreases whereas that for inhaled allergens increases with age in AD.[17] Immuno Solid-phase Allergen Chip (ISAC)-112 is a microarray-based *in vitro* test for assessing allergen-specific IgE in plasma. Prosperi et al. reported usefulness of ISAC testing in allergic airway disease but not in eczema in pediatric cohort.[18] However, in a recent pilot study, a potential role for ISAC testing was proposed in diagnosing sensitization and allergy in childhood AD.[19] *In vitro* testing for specific IgE remains more of a research tool, and routine use in AD is not indicated. Other blood investigations like peripheral blood eosinophilia and serum lactate dehydrogenase (LDH) measurement have also been proposed to indicate severity of AD. Mukai et al. have reported significant elevation of LDH in severe forms of AD, with LDH4 and LDH5 elevations having more prominent elevation in severe AD.[20] In addition to LDH, other serological parameters like soluble interleukin (IL)-2 receptor (sIL-2R), soluble CD23 (sCD23), and eosinophil cationic protein (ECP) elevations have also been seen in severe forms of AD compared to mild forms. However, these investigations still do not have a widespread clinical use due to inconsistent reporting in different studies.

Patch Test

Patch test is a standard investigation in patients suspected to have allergic contact dermatitis (ACD).[21] There is still no consensus whether the risk of ACD is elevated or decreased in patients with AD. While some studies have suggested that AD is a risk factor for ACD, others suggest that ACD is less frequent in AD patients than general population.[22,23] Some recent studies have indicated that the risk of ACD is elevated in patients with mild AD but decreased in severe AD.[23] Some of the studies regarding patch testing in AD and their findings are summarized in table 2. Recent clinical recommendations in 2016 by Chen et al. have given indications for performing patch testing in AD patients.[28] Patch test is done in AD if pattern is atypical or poorly responsive to topical therapy, if pattern is suggestive of CD, if there is therapy resistant hand eczema, in adolescent- or adult-onset AD, and in severe AD before starting systemic immunosuppressants. Patch testing is not recommended in case of well-controlled AD, recent flares, use of ultraviolet radiation in last 2 to 3 weeks, recent use of immunosuppressants, or in cases of inadequate patch test battery.

Atopy Patch Testing

Environmental factors like food and aeroallergens have been implicated in pathogenesis of AD. Allergy to food develops in first few years of life, whereas allergy to aeroallergens like mite and pollen develop later in childhood. Tests like atopy patch testing (APT) involves cutaneous application of intact allergen, followed by evaluation after 48 and 72 hours. In general, APT positivity for food as well as aeroallergens decreases with increasing age, possibly due to thicker

Table 2: Patch Testing in Atopic Dermatitis[23-27]	
Study	**Findings and conclusions**
Cronin and McFadden (1993)	Patch testing showed sensitivity to 1 or more allergens in 38% of existing atopic eczema patients, 53% of those with past eczema, 54% of those with mucous membrane eczema, and 50% of nonatopic patients. Since sensitization does occur in atopic dermatitis (AD), patch testing should be done in AD
Kapur et al. (2009)	Positivity of patch testing against dermatophagoides or house dust mite was statistically significant in AD as well as chronic eczema
Neodorost and Babineau (2010)	Number of positive patch test reaction in AD patients did not differ significantly from non-AD patients
Herro et al. (2011)	Children with AD, especially those with moderate to severe forms, have a significantly higher contact allergy than non-AD subjects and patch test is indicated in childhood AD
Thyssen et al. (2012)	Patients with severe AD have lower prevalence of contact sensitization compared to controls. However, mild to moderate AD does not suppress contact sensitization

skin or immune tolerance or both.[29] Atopy patch testing for food allergies is not standardized and most of the studies are with cow's milk, hen's egg, and wheat. Atopy patch testing for aeroallergens uses dust mites, animal dander, grass, and pollen. Atopy patch testing for aeroallergens is frequently positive in AD patients and is an additional diagnostic testing if flares occur on exposed areas on in certain seasons. The problem with APT testing for aeroallergens is that there is no gold standard for provocation testing and this also needs larger studies and standardization.[28,30,31]

Skin Prick Test

The diagnostic value of skin prick test in AD is controversial. While sensitization of patients to air borne and food borne allergens is common in AD, their role in flares or disease activity in AD is still not defined. A prick test for air-borne allergens can be recommended in AD in those patients who present with an airborne pattern of eczema on face, neck, flexures, and exposed parts of limbs. Skin prick test is useful to identify triggers for flares, particularly in moderate to severe cases.[32] Avoidance measures can then be undertaken in case of positive allergens. Prick tests can also be done for food allergies in adult AD patients but cross-reactions are frequent and avoidance of identified allergens has not always been successful in preventing the flare-ups of AD. Prick test can be done in chronic hand eczema if there is history suggestive of protein contact dermatitis.[33] According to some studies, skin prick test is less sensitive for food allergy in young children with AD.[34]

Skin Biopsy in Atopic Dermatitis

Routine skin biopsy is not indicated in AD. Skin biopsy can be performed only in specific conditions, including chronic AD, refractory to treatment, AD associated with erythroderma, morphological variant of prurigo and in conditions where AD needs to be differentiated from other skin diseases like psoriasis, skin eruptions, etc.[33] The histopathological findings in AD, as reported in studies, include acanthosis, parakeratosis, spongiosis, and exocytosis, with a chronic inflammatory infiltrate, mainly composed of lymphocytes, eosinophils, and mast cells. The same study reported IgE deposits in skin on direct immunofluorescence method.[35]

Vitamin D Testing in Atopic Dermatitis

In addition to its role in calcium metabolism, vitamin D also has immuno-modulating role and is associated with keratinocyte antimicrobial peptide production. Many studies have evaluated AD in vitamin D deficient individuals. In 2008, Oren et al. reported vitamin D deficient obese individuals to have a five-times higher risk of developing AD.[36] Peroni et al. reported higher levels of 25(OH) vitamin D levels in mild AD compared to moderate and severe forms, thereby implying that vitamin D deficiency may be related to severity of AD.[37] However, Back et al reported increased vitamin D intake to be correlated with increased risk of AD at 6 years of age.[38] Similarly, a cohort study in Finland has reported vitamin D supplementation in first year of life to be associated with higher incidence of atopy and allergic rhinitis at 31 years of age.[39] Chiu et al found no correlation with Vitamin D levels and severity of AD in children 1 to 16 years of age,[40] whereas a Korean study reported low vitamin D levels in adults to be associated with higher risk of AD.[41] Since the results are mixed and role of vitamin D supplementation in AD is still debatable, routine serum vitamin D estimation is not recommended.

NEWER BIOMARKERS IN ATOPIC DERMATITIS

Recent research has focused on identifying new biomarkers for AD, which may have a future role in identifying AD, determining disease severity and carry prognostic significance.

- Filaggrin (*FLG*) gene mutation: Filaggrin is an epidermal protein playing a key role in maintaining epidermal barrier function. Filaggrin gene mutations are commonly found in atopic disorders, including AD. These mutations occur in 30% of AD patients but all FLG mutation carriers do not develop AD.[42] Filaggrin gene mutations are more common in early onset AD as well as severe forms of AD. A meta-analysis has also shown a strong correlation of *FLG* gene mutation with atopic eczema.[43] Detection of FLG mutation thus may have a future role as both screening marker of early onset and severe AD, as well as in determining prognosis[44]

- Serum thymus and activation-regulated chemokine (TARC) is a chemokine belonging to T helper 2 (Th2) family, whose levels correlate most reliably with disease severity and activity as per a meta-analysis.[12] According to Tamaki et al., severity of AD can be classified as per serum TARC level (mild state: ≤700 pg/mL and moderate/severe state: >700 pg/mL).[45] It may also be possible to review patient education and treatments by using serum TARC levels as a parameter.[7] Abnormally high TARC levels correlate well with inflammation in AD and the levels fall significantly with topical anti-inflammatory therapy[46]

- Thymic stromal lymphopoietin (TSLP) plays a key role in Th2 type of inflammation through activation of dendritic cells. It also activates mast cells to promote cytokine production, thereby playing a role in development of eczematous lesions.[47] Elevated gene expression in lesional skin and elevated serum levels of TSLP have been reported in AD.[48] Epidermal TSLP protein expression has been reported to be a marker to identify at-risk children with AD.[49] Nygaard et al. have reported significant elevation of TSLP, IL-31, and IL-33 levels in AD patients but not with soluble ST2 levels.[50] The same study reported inverse relationship between IL-33 and sST2 levels. Periostin (POSTN) is a factor induced by Th-2 related cytokines like IL-4 and IL-13. It has been postulated to play a role as mediator in amplifying and maintaining Th2 type inflammation in AD. Kou et al. have reported significantly higher levels of periostin in AD patients compared to controls, with higher levels in extrinsic AD than intrinsic.[51] Sung et al. have reported association of serum periostin levels with severity and chronicity in childhood AD.[52] A recent study by Uysal et al. reported higher serum levels of TARC, TSLP, and serum periostin in childhood AD. Serum periostin levels showed a positive modest correlation with age and duration with AD. The authors concluded that while serum periostin may be used as a marker to predict atopy and chronicity, serum TSLP and TARC can predict severity in AD[53]

- Measurement of specific subset of T-cells is also under consideration as potential biomarkers for AD. Cutaneous lymphocyte-associated antigen positive (CLA+) T-cells are the major T cell population in AD lesions. As per a recent study, elevated levels of circulating CLA+ T cells may be a surrogate marker of inflammation and disease activity in AD patients and may obviate the need for skin biopsy for immune phenotyping in select cases of severe AD.[54] Recently, Szabó et al. reported increased number of circulating IL-21 producing follicular T helper cells in children with AD compared to adult patients[55]

- Other potential screening biomarkers in AD that have been reported in various studies include elevated infantile lymphotoxin-α, elevated cord blood IgE levels, and detection of specific FceRI-b genotypes during pregnancy, which may predict childhood AD[56]
- During immunoglobulin synthesis, light chains are produced in excess over heavy chains. Since light chains have a shorter half-life and since the natural course of AD is relapsing and remitting, Ig-free light chains (Ig-FLCs) levels are theoretically more suitable as a biomarker than total serum IgE for disease severity. Serum kappa-Ig-FLCs have been reported to be significantly elevated in children with AD compared to controls.[57] The elevation is significantly more in severe forms of childhood AD than mild forms but the correlation of Ig-FLCs with adult onset AD was reported to be absent[58]
- In a recent study evaluating the levels of cytokines in AD, blood levels of specific cytokines and anti-staphylococcus enterotoxin A and B immunoglobulin E (anti-SEA and anti-SEB) levels were assessed in AD patients. The authors reported significant correlation between blood levels of Th1, regulatory T cells (Treg), anti-SEB, and APC cytokines like IL-18 and IL-23 with various clinical signs of AD[59]
- The skin density of *Staphylococcus aureus* has been proposed as another prognostic investigation. Tauber et al. reported correlation between skin density of *S. aureus* on both lesional and nonlesional areas with disease severity scores in AD patients[60]
- Itching is a significant morbidity in AD and a cause of decreased quality of life in AD. Serum IL-31 is considered a marker of pruritus and some recent research has shown promising results in correlation between serum IL-31 levels and disease activity, although further studies are still awaited before definite conclusions can be made[61]
- Indoleamine 2,3-dioxygenase-1 has been proposed to be a marker for eczema herpeticum form of AD.[62] Additional markers that might be useful in future in AD patients include serum cutaneous T-cell attracting chemokine, macrophage-derived chemokine, serum and hair mean zinc levels, sE-selectin.[12,41,63] More research is needed though, to comment upon their exact role in AD.

INVESTIGATIONS TO ASSESS SKIN BARRIER FUNCTION

- Transepidermal water loss (TEWL) measures water diffusion through the skin *in vivo* and is considered an important functional parameter to assess skin barrier integrity.[64] Raised TEWL has been reported to precede the development of clinical lesions in AD.[65] Kelleher et al. have reported in a 2015 study that measurement of TEWL with a validated open chamber method like Tewameter TM 300 on day 2 of life can predict development of AD at 1 year of age.[66] Transepidermal water loss measurement can, therefore, be a potential marker to identify neonates at-risk for AD. Such neonates can then be followed up and emollients started at an early stage

- Raman microspectroscopy: Raman spectroscopy is a noninvasive technique based upon inelastic light scattering (Raman scattering) of monochromatic light, which provides information regarding skin composition, including water content and amino acid composition. Raman spectroscopy has been shown to permit rapid and accurate stratification of AD associated with FLG mutations.[67] Verzeaux et al. used confocal Raman microspectroscopy (CRS) to reveal altered lipid status and impaired barrier function in stratum corneum of AD patients.[68] A recent study using CRS revealed lower water and natural moisturizing factor content in AD patients with *FLG* mutations but not in those with sensitive skin.[69] Confocal Raman microspectroscopy remains a potential noninvasive tool to identify skin barrier disruption in AD.

INVESTIGATIONS TO ASSESS COMORBIDITIES IN ATOPIC DERMATITIS

Since AD is associated with multiple comorbidities, it is considered more as a systemic disease than simply a dermatological disorder. Comorbidities reported in AD patients range from association with other atopic disorders like allergic rhinitis, food allergies and asthma, increased risk of infections, malignancy (including lymphomas), cardiovascular and neuropsychiatric disorders.[70] A patient with AD, therefore, needs to be followed up and evaluated for these comorbidities as well.

CONCLUSION

Diagnosis of AD is primarily clinical, with little role of any diagnostic investigations. Blood investigations like IgE, LDH measurement, although shown promise in some studies, other studies have reported mixed results. Investigations like patch testing, prick tests, and skin biopsy are recommended only in specific circumstances. Recent advancements have opened up the role of various potential biomarkers, not only in screening, but also to prognosticate and document disease activity in AD. Larger studies are needed before specific recommendations of these biomarkers can be made in AD.

Editor's Comment

Investigations in atopic dermatitis (AD) can have a role in diagnosis, classification, and prognosis. Investigations are also important in identifying the triggers of AD and in assessing comorbidities. This article reiterates the role of Immunoglobulin E (IgE), patch test and future biomarkers to supplement clinical diagnosis of atopic dermatitis.

Rashmi Sarkar

REFERENCES

1. Eichenfield LF, Tom WL, Chamlin SL, et al. Guidelines of care for the management of atopic dermatitis: section 1. Diagnosis and assessment of atopic dermatitis. *J Am Acad Dermatol.* 2014;70(2):338-51.
2. Williams HC, Burney PG, Hay RJ, et al. The U.K. Working Party's Diagnostic Criteria for Atopic Dermatitis. I. Derivation of a minimum set of discriminators for atopic dermatitis. *Br J Dermatol.* 1994;131(3):383-96.
3. Williams HC, Burney PG, Strachan D, et al. The U.K. Working Party's Diagnostic Criteria for Atopic Dermatitis. II. Observer variation of clinical diagnosis and signs of atopic dermatitis. *Br J Dermatol.* 1994;131(3):397-405.
4. Firooz A, Davoudi SM, Farahmand AN, et al. Validation of the diagnostic criteria for atopic dermatitis. *Arch Dermatol.* 1999;135(5):514-6.
5. De D, Kanwar AJ, Handa S. Comparative efficacy of Hanifin and Rajka's criteria and the UK working party's diagnostic criteria in diagnosis of atopic dermatitis in a hospital setting in North India. *J Eur Acad Dermatol Venereol.* 2006;20(7):853-9.
6. Kang KF, Tian RM. Criteria for atopic dermatitis in a Chinese population. *Acta Derm Venereol Suppl (Stockh).* 1989;144:26-7.
7. Saeki H, Nakahara T, Tanaka A, et al. Clinical practice guidelines for the management of atopic dermatitis. *J Dermatol.* 2016;43(10):1117-45.
8. Bos JD, Van Leent EJ, Sillevis Smitt JH. The millennium criteria for the diagnosis of atopic dermatitis. *Exp Dermatol.* 1998;7(4):132-8.
9. Ott H, Stanzel S, Ocklenburg C, et al. Total serum IgE as a parameter to differentiate between intrinsic and extrinsic atopic dermatitis in children. *Acta Derm Venereol.* 2009;89(3):257-61.
10. Kiiski V, Karlsson O, Remitz A, et al. High serum total IgE predicts poor long-term outcome in atopic dermatitis. *Acta Derm Venereol.* 2015;95(8):943-7.
11. Glatz M, Buchner M, von Bartenwerffer W, et al. Malassezia spp.-specific immunoglobulin E level is a marker for severity of atopic dermatitis in adults. *Acta Derm Venereol.* 2015;95(2):191-6.
12. Thijs J, Krastev T, Weidinger S, et al. Biomarkers for atopic dermatitis: A systematic review and meta-analysis. *Curr Opin Allergy Clin Immunol.* 2015;15(5):453-60.
13. Banerjee S, Resch Y, Chen KW, et al. Der p 11 is a major allergen for house dust mite-allergic patients suffering from atopic dermatitis. *J Invest Dermatol.* 2015;135(1):102-9.
14. Mittermann I, Wikberg G, Johansson C, et al. IgE sensitization profiles differ between adult patients with severe and moderate atopic dermatitis. *PLoS One.* 2016;11(5):e0156077.
15. Ohman S, Johansson SG. Allergen-specific IgE in atopic dermatitis. *Acta Derm Venereol.* 1974;54(4):283-90.
16. Takahashi I, Akiyama T, Yamaura H, et al. Evaluation of RAST in atopic dermatitis. *J Dermatol.* 1977;4(6):217-21.
17. Rudzki E, Litewska D. RAST and PRIST in children with atopic dermatitis. *Dermatologica.* 1990;180(2):82-5.

18. Prosperi MC, Belgrave D, Buchan I, et al. Challenges in interpreting allergen microarrays in relation to clinical symptoms: A machine learning approach. *Pediatr Allergy Immunol.* 2014;25(1):71-9.

19. Foong RX, Roberts G, Fox AT, et al. Pilot study: assessing the clinical diagnosis of allergy in atopic children using a microarray assay in addition to skin prick testing and serum specific IgE. *Clin Mol Allergy.* 2016;14:8.

20. Mukai H, Noguchi T, Kamimura K, et al. Significance of elevated serum LDH (lactate dehydrogenase) activity in atopic dermatitis. *J Dermatol.* 1990;17(8):477-81.

21. Fonacier L, Bernstein DI, Pacheco K, et al. Contact dermatitis: a practice parameter-update 2015. *J Allergy Clin Immunol Pract.* 2015;3(3 Suppl):S1-39.

22. Whitmore SE. Should atopic individuals be patch tested? *Dermatol Clin.* 1994;12(3):491-9.

23. Thyssen JP, Johansen JD, Linneberg A, et al. The association between contact sensitization and atopic disease by linkage of a clinical database and a nationwide patient registry. *Allergy.* 2012;67(9):1157-64.

24. Kapur C, Shenoi SD, Prabhu SS, et al. Patch testing with dermatophagoides and its correlation with chronic eczema and atopic dermatitis. *Indian J Dermatol.* 2009;54(3):243-6.

25. Herro EM, Matiz C, Sullivan K, et al. Frequency of contact allergens in pediatric patients with atopic dermatitis. *J Clin Aesthet Dermatol.* 2011;4(11):39-41.

26. Nedorost ST, Babineau D. Patch testing in atopic dermatitis. *Dermatitis.* 2010;21(5):251-4.

27. Cronin E, McFadden JP. Patients with atopic eczema do become sensitized to contact allergens. *Contact Dermatitis.* 1993;28(4):225-8.

28. Chen JK, Jacob SE, Nedorost ST, et al. A pragmatic approach to patch testing atopic dermatitis patients: Clinical recommendations based on expert consensus opinion. *Dermatitis.* 2016;27(4):186-92.

29. Jurakic Toncic R, Lipozencic J. Role and significance of atopy patch test. *Acta Dermatovenerol Croat.* 2010;18(1):38-55.

30. Kerschenlohr K, Darsow U, Burgdorf WH, et al. Lessons from atopy patch testing in atopic dermatitis. *Curr Allergy Asthma Rep.* 2004;4(4):285-9.

31. Turjanmaa K, Darsow U, Niggemann B, et al. EAACI/GA2LEN position paper: present status of the atopy patch test. *Allergy.* 2006;61(12):1377-84.

32. Caffarelli C, Dondi A, Povesi Dascola C, et al. Skin prick test to foods in childhood atopic eczema: Pros and cons. *Ital J Pediatr.* 2013;39:48.

33. Silvestre Salvador JF, Romero-Perez D, Encabo-Duran B. Atopic dermatitis in adults: A diagnostic challenge. *J Investig Allergol Clin Immunol.* 2017;27(2):78-88.

34. Stromberg L. Diagnostic accuracy of the atopy patch test and the skin-prick test for the diagnosis of food allergy in young children with atopic eczema/dermatitis syndrome. *Acta Paediatr.* 2002;91(10):1044-9.

35. Piloto Valdes L, Gomez Echevarria AH, Valdes Sanchez AF, et al. Atopic dermatitis. Findings of skin biopsies. *Allergol Immunopathol (Madr).* 1990;18(6):321-4.

36. Oren E, Banerji A, Camargo CA, Jr. Vitamin D and atopic disorders in an obese population screened for vitamin D deficiency. *J Allergy Clin Immunol.* 2008;121(2):533-4.

37. Peroni DG, Piacentini GL, Cametti E, et al. Correlation between serum 25-hydroxyvitamin D levels and severity of atopic dermatitis in children. *Br J Dermatol.* 2011;164(5):1078-82.

38. Back O, Blomquist HK, Hernell O, et al. Does vitamin D intake during infancy promote the development of atopic allergy? *Acta Derm Venereol.* 2009;89(1):28-32.

39. Hypponen E, Sovio U, Wjst M, et al. Infant vitamin D supplementation and allergic conditions in adulthood: northern Finland birth cohort 1966. *Ann N Y Acad Sci.* 2004;1037:84-95.

40. Chiu YE, Havens PL, Siegel DH, et al. Serum 25-hydroxyvitamin D concentration does not correlate with atopic dermatitis severity. *J Am Acad Dermatol.* 2013;69(1):40-6.

41. Cheng HM, Kim S, Park GH, et al. Low vitamin D levels are associated with atopic dermatitis, but not allergic rhinitis, asthma, or IgE sensitization, in the adult Korean population. *J Allergy Clin Immunol.* 2014;133(4):1048-55.

42. Weidinger S, O'Sullivan M, Illig T, et al. Filaggrin mutations, atopic eczema, hay fever, and asthma in children. *J Allergy Clin Immunol.* 2008;121(5):1203-9 e1.

43. van den Oord RA, Sheikh A. Filaggrin gene defects and risk of developing allergic sensitisation and allergic disorders: Systematic review and meta-analysis. *BMJ*. 2009;339.
44. Barker JN, Palmer CN, Zhao Y, et al. Null mutations in the filaggrin gene (FLG) determine major susceptibility to early-onset atopic dermatitis that persists into adulthood. *J Invest Dermatol*. 2007;127(3):564-7.
45. Tamaki K, Kakinuma T, Saeki H, et al. Serum levels of CCL17/TARC in various skin diseases. *J Dermatol*. 2006;33(4):300-2.
46. Yasukochi Y, Nakahara T, Abe T, et al. Reduction of serum TARC levels in atopic dermatitis by topical anti-inflammatory treatments. *Asian Pac J Allergy Immunol*. 2014;32(3):240-5.
47. Allakhverdi Z, Comeau MR, Jessup HK, et al. Thymic stromal lymphopoietin is released by human epithelial cells in response to microbes, trauma, or inflammation and potently activates mast cells. *J Exp Med*. 2007;204(2):253-8.
48. Alysandratos KD, Angelidou A, Vasiadi M, et al. Increased affected skin gene expression and serum levels of thymic stromal lymphopoietin in atopic dermatitis. *Ann Allergy Asthma Immunol*. 2010;105(5):403-4.
49. Kim J, Kim BE, Lee J, et al. Epidermal thymic stromal lymphopoietin predicts the development of atopic dermatitis during infancy. *J Allergy Clin Immunol*. 2016;137(4):1282-5 e1-4.
50. Nygaard U, Hvid M, Johansen C, et al. TSLP, IL-31, IL-33 and sST2 are new biomarkers in endophenotypic profiling of adult and childhood atopic dermatitis. *J Eur Acad Dermatol Venereol*. 2016;30(11):1930-8.
51. Kou K, Okawa T, Yamaguchi Y, et al. Periostin levels correlate with disease severity and chronicity in patients with atopic dermatitis. *Br J Dermatol*. 2014;171(2):283-91.
52. Sung M, Lee KS, Ha EG, et al. An association of periostin levels with the severity and chronicity of atopic dermatitis in children. *Pediatr Allergy Immunol*. 2017;28(6):543-50.
53. Uysal P, Birtekocak F, Karul AB. The relationship between serum TARC, TSLP and POSTN levels and childhood atopic dermatitis. *Clin Lab*. 2017;63(7):1071-7.
54. Czarnowicki T, Santamaria-Babí LF, Guttman-Yassky E. Circulating CLA+ T cells in atopic dermatitis and their possible role as peripheral biomarkers. *Allergy*. 2017;72(3):366-72.
55. Szabo K, Gaspar K, Dajnoki Z, et al. Expansion of circulating follicular T helper cells associates with disease severity in childhood atopic dermatitis. *Immunol Lett*. 2017;189:101-8.
56. Wen HJ, Wang YJ, Lin YC, et al. Prediction of atopic dermatitis in 2-yr-old children by cord blood IgE, genetic polymorphisms in cytokine genes, and maternal mentality during pregnancy. *Pediatr Allergy Immunol*. 2011;22(7):695-703.
57. Kayserova J, Capkova S, Skalicka A, et al. Serum immunoglobulin free light chains in severe forms of atopic dermatitis. *Scand J Immunol*. 2010;71(4):312-6.
58. Thijs JL, Knipping K, Bruijnzeel-Koomen CA, et al. Immunoglobulin free light chains in adult atopic dermatitis patients do not correlate with disease severity. *Clin Transl Allergy*. 2016;6:44.
59. Hon K, Tsang K, Kung J, et al. Clinical signs, Staphylococcus and atopic eczema-related seromarkers. *Molecules*. 2017;22(2):291.
60. Tauber M, Balica S, Hsu CY, et al. Staphylococcus aureus density on lesional and nonlesional skin is strongly associated with disease severity in atopic dermatitis. *J Allergy Clin Immunol*. 2016;137(4):1272-4 e1-3.
61. Raap U, Weissmantel S, Gehring M, et al. IL-31 significantly correlates with disease activity and Th2 cytokine levels in children with atopic dermatitis. *Pediatr Allergy Immunol*. 2012;23(3):285-8.
62. Staudacher A, Hinz T, Novak N, et al. Exaggerated IDO1 expression and activity in Langerhans cells from patients with atopic dermatitis upon viral stimulation: A potential predictive biomarker for high risk of Eczema herpeticum. *Allergy*. 2015;70(11):1432-9.
63. Kim JE, Yoo SR, Jeong MG, et al. Hair zinc levels and the efficacy of oral zinc supplementation in patients with atopic dermatitis. *Acta Derm Venereol*. 2014;94(5):558-62.
64. Addor FA, Aoki V. Barreira cutânea na dermatite atópica. *Anais Brasileiros de Dermatologia*. 2010;85:184-94.
65. Flohr C, England K, Radulovic S, et al. Filaggrin loss-of-function mutations are associated with early-onset eczema, eczema severity and transepidermal water loss at 3 months of age. *Br J Dermatol*. 2010;163(6): 1333-6.

66. Kelleher M, Dunn-Galvin A, Hourihane JO, et al. Skin barrier dysfunction measured by transepidermal water loss at 2 days and 2 months predates and predicts atopic dermatitis at 1 year. *J Allergy Clin Immunol.* 2015; 135(4):930-5.e1.

67. O'Regan GM, Kemperman PM, Sandilands A, et al. Raman profiles of the stratum corneum define 3 filaggrin genotype-determined atopic dermatitis endophenotypes. *J Allergy Clin Immunol.* 2010;126(3):574-80.e1.

68. Verzeaux L, Vyumvuhore R, Boudier D, et al. Atopic skin: In vivo Raman identification of global molecular signature, a comparative study with healthy skin. *Exp Dermatol.* 2017. [Epub before print].

69. Richters RJH, Falcone D, Uzunbajakava NE, et al. Sensitive skin: Assessment of the skin barrier using confocal raman microspectroscopy. *Skin Pharmacol Physiol.* 2017;30(1):1-12.

70. Brunner PM, Silverberg JI, Guttman-Yassky E, et al. Increasing comorbidities suggest that atopic dermatitis is a systemic disorder. *J Invest Dermatol.* 2017;137(1):18-25.

World Clin Dermatol. 2018;4(1):59-68.

Atopic Dermatitis
Treatment Topical Therapy

María E Abad MD, *Margarita Larralde MD PhD

Department of Dermatology, Aleman Hospital; Department of Pediatric Dermatology
Ramos Mejía Hospital, Buenos Aires, Argentina

ABSTRACT

Atopic dermatitis (AD) is a chronic inflammatory skin disease characterized by pruritus, xerosis, and relapsing eczemas in a typical distribution. Most AD patients have a mild to moderate disease which can be successfully managed with basic skin care measures, avoiding irritants and triggering factors, regular use of moisturizers, and topical pharmacological treatment. First-line topical therapy includes topical corticosteroids (TC). Topical calcineurin inhibitors (TCI) are considered a second-line option acting as a steroid-sparing agent, particularly in high sensitive areas (face, eyelids, skin folds, and genitalia). In addition, TCI are preferred in case of steroid-induced skin atrophy, recalcitrant lesions to TC, long-term uninterrupted TC use, and steroid-phobia. Proactive treatment consists of topical application of an anti-inflammatory agent (TC or TCI) once active lesions have been controlled to prevent, delay and decrease disease flares. Finally, new emerging therapies with different mechanism of action are currently being developed, including phosphodiesterase-4 inhibitors (crisaborole) and Janus kinase inhibitors (topical tofacitinib).

INTRODUCTION

Atopic dermatitis (AD) is a common chronic and inflammatory disease, characterized by pruritus, xerosis, and relapsing eczematous lesions in a typical distribution. Its prevalence is estimated between 10 and 30% in children and 10% in adults. Disease onset occurs typically during the first year of life in 65% of the cases, and before the age of 5 in 85% of affected children.[1,2]

---

*Corresponding author
Email: doctoralarralde@gmail.com

The aim of therapeutic strategies of AD is to control symptoms, to prevent relapses, and to improve quality of life of the patients and their families. Management of AD includes interventions to restore epidermal barrier function as well as to suppress the inflammatory response.

DISCUSSION

Most of AD patients have a mild disease that can be successfully managed with basic skin care measures, including bathing practices, moisturizers, and avoiding irritants and triggering factors. Education of the patient and their parents/caregivers is an important strategy to improve treatment adherence.

Commonly Used Topical Treatment

Topical treatment is the first-line approach of AD, either alone or associated with systemic therapies in the case of severe disease. Topical management includes moisturizers, dilute bleach baths, and anti-inflammatory medications—topical corticosteroids and topical calcineurin inhibitors.

Moisturizers

Skin barrier dysfunction is thought to have an important role in allergic sensitization, initiation, and progression of AD. It is characterized by xerosis and an increase of transepidermal water loss. One of the most important intervention to repair the damaged epidermal barrier is the regular use of moisturizers. Frequent moisturization hydrate the skin, alleviate the discomfort associated with xerosis and pruritus, reduce the number of flares and prolong the time to flare, and finally decrease the need of topical corticosteroids. Therefore, emollients are the first-line approach for the management of AD.[3-5]

Moisturizers should be applied at least once daily within 3 minutes after bathing to favor skin hydration. Although there is a lack of evidence regarding the optimal frequency to apply the emollient, it is recommended to use them liberally.

Recently, it has been demonstrated that the use of moisturizers in newborns at high risk for AD, at least once daily starting within the first three weeks of life, can prevent the development of the disease. The authors propose that moisturizers improve epidermal barrier dysfunction and reduce skin permeability, preventing allergic sensitization.[6]

Bleach Baths

Staphylococcus aureus overgrowth on AD skin—with or without cutaneous infection—has been associated with increased relapses and severity of the disease, in part due to the production of toxins that act as superantigens.[3,7] Patients with moderate to severe AD and recurrent infections may benefit with the use of dilute bleach baths. It has been demonstrated the antistaphylococcal activity of sodium hypochlorite, including methicillin resistant *S. aureus*, by producing irreversible aggregation of essential bacterial proteins.[8]

To obtain a final concentration of 0.005% add 4 ounces (1/2 cup) of common household bleach (sodium hypochlorite 6%) to a standard bathtub full of warm water. Patients are told to soak neck down for 5–10 minutes, then rinse off with normal tap water and finally apply emollients to prevent dryness and irritation, twice to three times a week.[7,9]

Although dilute bleach baths are well tolerated, cheap, and easily accessible, further investigation is needed to assess the impact of this practice on AD patients.

Topical Corticosteroids

Topical corticosteroids (TC) are the mainstay of anti-inflammatory treatment of AD since their introduction in the 1950s. They are classified according to their potency into seven groups, ranging from class I, which are the most potent to class VII, the lowest potent (Table 1).[3,10-13] Potency is based on vasoconstrictor assays, and has a variation of 1,800 times between the lowest and the highest potency.[10,14] Topical steroids are available in diverse vehicles, including ointment, cream, lotion, gel, foam, and spray, which are suitable for different areas of the skin. Ointments have a higher relative potency because of their occlusive effect and are less likely to produce burning or stinging symptoms when applied on eroded skin.[10,13]

The American Academy of Dermatology recommends the use of TC for reactive and proactive AD management.[3]

Mechanism of Action

Steroids bind cytoplasmic receptors and form a complex that translocate into the nucleus of a targeted cell and induce activation of steroid responsive genes. The pharmacological activity of TC includes:

- Suppression of proinflammatory cytokines [interleukins (IL-1α, IL-1β, IL-2), tumor necrosis factor (TNF), granulocyte-monocyte colony stimulating factor (GM-CSF)]
- Induction of anti-inflammatory proteins (vasocortin, vasoregulin, lipocortin)
- Decrease the number and activity of immune cells, including neutrophils, lymphocytes, monocytes, and Langerhans cells
- Reduction of the production of structural cytokines.[3,4,12]

Table 1: Topical corticosteroids: Classification regarding relative potency

Class I: Superpotent/highest potency
- Clobetasol propionate 0.05% ointment, cream, foam, solution
- Diflorasone diacetate 0.05% ointment
- Halobetasol propionate 0.05% ointment, cream

Class II: High potency
- Betamethasone dipropionate 0.05% ointment, cream, gel, foam, solution
- Diflorasone diacetate 0.05% cream
- Fluocinonide 0.05% ointment, cream, gel, solution
- Mometasone furoate 0.1% ointment
- Triamcinolone acetonide 0.5% ointment, cream

Class III: Moderate potency
- Betamethasone valerate 0.1% ointment
- Fluticasone propionate 0.005% ointment
- Mometasone furoate 0.1% ointment
- Triamcinolone acetonide 0.1% ointment

Class IV: Moderate potency
- Betamethasone valerate 0.1% foam
- Fluticasone propionate 0.005% cream
- Hydrocortisone valerate 0.2% ointment
- Mometasone furoate 0.1% cream
- Triamcinolone acetonide 0.1% cream

Class V: Lower-moderate potency
- Hydrocortisone butyrate 0.1% ointment, cream, solution
- Hydrocortisone valerate 0.2% cream
- Prednicarbate 0.1% cream

Class VI: Low potency
- Desonide 0.005% ointment, cream, gel, foam
- Fluocinolone acetonide 0.01% cream, solution

Class VII: Lowest potency
- Dexamethasone 0.1% cream
- Hydrocortisone acetate 0.5–1% ointment, cream
- Hydrocortisone hydrochloride 0.25–2.5% ointment, cream, lotion, solution

Efficacy

The efficacy of TC for the treatment of both acute and chronic lesions of AD has been demonstrated. They are also effective in reducing pruritus.[3]

Dosage/Regimens

The potency and vehicle choice of TC depends on a variety of factors such as age of the patient, previous treatment, lesion site, and disease severity. Low-potency

TC are useful in the face, neck, and folds and are a good option in case of mild AD, whereas moderate-potency TC are the best choice for the trunk and limbs and in case of moderate acute flare. Short courses of superpotent or high-potency steroids are reserved for the treatment of chronic and lichenified lesions of AD.[10,11,13] Topical steroids should be applied as a thin layer at night during acute flares until the treated area is clear.[2]

Adverse Effects

Potential side effects are related to the potency and the length of TC used. Cutaneous/local side effects occur at the site of application and include skin atrophy, striae, purpura, telangiectasia, hypertrichosis, depigmentation, delay in wound healing, folliculitis, periorificial dermatitis, acneiform eruption, and secondary infection, or exacerbation of a previous infection.[3,14,15] There is also a potential risk of developing cataracts or glaucoma when used at periocular area.[3,10] Allergic contact dermatitis may be produced by the steroid molecule or other ingredient of the vehicle. It should be suspected if lesions fail to respond or worsen despite of adequate TC treatment. Patch testing can help to establish the etiology of the allergen.[3,14]

Generalized side effects from systemic absorption are rare and related to the use of high-potency TC, applied over a wide cutaneous area for a long period of time. Systemic adverse events include hypothalamic-pituitary axis suppression, hyperglycemia, hypertension, femoral avascular head necrosis, and growth retardation.[3,13,16]

Topical Calcineurin Inhibitors

Topical calcineurin inhibitors (TCIs) are macrolides produced by *Streptomyces* species. They are nonsteroidal immunomodulators that became an alternative to TC which are the first-line therapy for AD. They have been used as topical immunosuppressive agents since their approval in 2000. Tacrolimus ointment 0.1–0.03% is approved for moderate to severe AD and pimecrolimus cream 1% for mild to moderate AD.

Mechanism of Action

Topical calcineurin inhibitors inhibit the catalytic function of calcineurin, the dephosphorylation of the nuclear factor of activated T cells (NFAT), blocking the transport of NFAT to the cell nucleus and finally inhibiting the transcription of proinflammatory cytokine genes (IL-2,IL-3, IL-4, IL-12, TNF, IFN-γ, GM-CSF).[2,4,17] Apart from the inactivation of T lymphocytes, TCI also inhibit the activation of other key effector cells involved in the pathogenesis of AD, including mastocytes, keratinocytes, and dendritic cells.[3,4,14]

Dosage/Regimens

Twice daily application of pimecrolimus 1% cream and tacrolimus 0.03% ointment are approved for AD in individuals age 2 years and older, whereas tacrolimus 0.1% is indicated in patients older than 15 years. Off label use of pimecrolimus 1% or tacrolimus 0.03% can be recommended for patients younger than 2 years of age.[3,16]

Efficacy

Both tacrolimus and pimecrolimus have demonstrated their efficacy in short term (3–12 weeks) and intermittent long term (3–12 weeks) treatments.[4,14] Topical calcineurin inhibitors are useful as a steroid-sparing agent, particularly in highly sensitive areas like the face, eyelids, skin folds, and genitalia, as they do not induce skin atrophy. Additionally, TCI are preferred in case of steroid-induced skin atrophy, recalcitrant lesions to TC, long-term uninterrupted TC use and steroid-phobia.[3,14,16]

Adverse Effects

The most common side effects are a localized short-live (minutes to hours) burning or stinging sensation and pruritus at the application site that decrease with continuous use (3–7 days). Furthermore, less frequent localized adverse events are skin erythema, folliculitis, allergic contact dermatitis, rosacea-like granulomatous reaction, perioral dermatitis, and local erythema after alcohol intake.[3,12,17] Although it has not been demonstrated, an increase in the occurrence of cutaneous infections, patients, and parents should be advised of this theoretical risk. Topical calcineurin inhibitors should be avoided in patients with ichthyosiform erythroderma like Netherton syndrome because of their increased percutaneous absorption that can induce systemic adverse effects.[15] Based on the well-known risk of malignancy with oral calcineurin inhibitors and on rare case reports of skin cancer and lymphoma in patients treated with TCI, although a causal relationship has not been demonstrated, the Food and Drug Administration placed a black-box warning in 2006. To date, there are numerous clinical studies published which demonstrate that systemic exposure to TCIs is minimal and transient and conclude that there is no evidence of a clear relationship between the use of TCI and an increase risk of malignancy.[3,17-19]

Topical Corticosteroids and Topical Calcineurin Inhibitors: Combination Therapy

In clinical practice TC and TCI are often used in combination—concomitantly or sequentially. A short course (4–7 days) of medium to high-potency topical steroids are better to control an acute flare of AD, followed by TCI acting as a steroid-sparing agent. Given the higher potency of TC to control the AD symptoms and the capacity of reducing the local adverse effects of TCI, TC are preferred to be used first in a step-wise therapy approach.[3,11,12]

Proactive Therapy

Reactive treatment refers to treating only active AD lesions with TC and/or TCI, whereas proactive treatment consists of topical application of an anti-inflammatory agent once active lesions have been controlled. It has been demonstrated that proactive approach not only prevent, delay, and decrease disease flares, but also reduce the amount of anti-inflammatory agent, the treatment days required to achieve remission of the exacerbation and improve the quality of life.[12,14] The rationale for the use of proactive treatment is based on the persistence of epidermal barrier dysfunction and subclinical inflammation in non-active lesions. Intermittent use of once daily TC (1–2 times/week) or once daily TCI (2–3 times/week) during remission to areas previously affected along with emollients is useful in those patients who suffer frequent relapses at the same site.[3,4,11,12]

Wet-wrap Therapy

Wet-wrap therapy (WWT) is an efficacious treatment for ambulatory or hospitalized patients with moderate to severe AD with acute and/or recalcitrant flares. The method used for WWT consists in the application of moisturizers or TC over the eczema lesions covered by a wet layer of dressing (tubular bandage or gauze), followed by a second dry bandage. The wrap can be worn under ordinary or nightwear clothes, and can be used during various to 24 hours at a time.[3,14,20,21] There are several proposed mechanisms of action: Moisture increases skin hydration and penetration of TC, helping to restore the damaged epidermal barrier and reducing the pruritus. In addition, wet dressings are a physical obstacle against scratching, breaking the itch-scratch cycle, improve sleep, and help to debride crusts, scales, and exudate.[14,20] Adverse effects of WWT include folliculitis, increase skin infections, and discomfort during treatment. Additionally, when used with TC under occlusion, there is an increased risk of hypothalamic-pituitary-adrenal axis suppression. Therefore, the duration of WWT with TC should be limited to a few days (7–14 days) using a low to medium potency topical steroid. Creams are preferred instead of ointments because they are less occlusive.[3,20,21]

Novel and Upcoming Topical Therapies

Current AD topical treatment has not changed for more than 15 years and is associated in some cases with certain limitations, including restrictions on their use on specific body sites and deficient efficacy. New emerging therapies with different mechanism of action are currently being developed.

Phosphodiesterase-4 Inhibitors

Phosphodiesterase (PDE) is an intracellular enzyme that selectively inhibits the activity of cyclic adenosine monophosphate (cAMP). The inactivation of PDE-4 increases intracellular cAMP levels, which suppress the activity of inflammatory signaling pathways like NK-κB among others, involved in proinflammatory cytokine production (IL-2, IL-4, IL-5, IL-10, IL-13, TNF-α, and IFN-γ).[2,22]

Crisaborole (previously known as AN2728) is a low-molecular-weight selective topical PDE-4 inhibitor with an efficient skin penetration into the epidermis and dermis and minimal systemic exposure attributable to its rapid metabolism into inactive metabolites. Twice daily application of crisaborole ointment 2% have been approved in the United States for the topical treatment of mild to moderate atopic dermatitis in patients aged 2 years and older. Crisaborole efficacy has been demonstrated with decrease in disease and pruritus severity and improvement of AD signs like erythema, exudation, excoriation, induration, and lichenification. Clinical studies have demonstrated a good safety profile in the short-term (28 days) and long-term (up to 52 weeks) therapy. The most frequently reported adverse effects were pruritus, dermatitis, and application site pain. Further long-term studies, including children under 2 years of age, are expected in the future.[2,12,16,22,23]

Janus Kinase Inhibitors

The Janus kinases (JAK)-signal transducer and activator of transcription (JAK-STAT) pathway is used by numerous cytokines and other molecules (IL-4, IL-12, IL-23, thymic stromal lymphopoietin, IFN-γ) for signal transduction from the cell membrane to the nucleus. Janus kinases are a group of four intracellular tyrosine kinases—JAK1, JAK2, JAK3, and tyrosine kinase 2 (Tyk2).[12,24-26] The small size of JAK inhibitors made them suitable for topical use.

Tofacitinib is a potent inhibitor of JAK-3 and at a lower level of JAK1 and JAK2, leading to the blockage of signaling through several cytokine receptors, including IL-4, IL-13, and IL-31 (pruritus specific interleukin) and additionally decreasing inflammation.[2,26] Tofacitinib ointment 1% twice daily in adults with mild to moderate AD was compared with vehicle for four weeks. The study showed significant clinical improvement and decreased pruritus with an acceptable safety profile in the tofacitinib group.[26]

Although JAK inhibitors represent a promising new treatment modality, further studies are needed to determine the efficacy, long-term safety, and administration regimen.

CONCLUSION

Topical therapies as well as skin care measures and education of patients and parents/caregivers are the most important strategies to achieve treatment success. Although safety concerns related to sensitive areas or long-term use, TC remain the first-line option for AD. The increasing understanding of AD pathophysiology is critical for developing more specific targeted therapies.

Editor's Comment

Topical therapy is very important in management of atopic dermatitis in children. Time tested remedies like emollients, wet wrap therapy, and bleach baths are important in decreasing severity of the disease. Recently, there is a lot of excitement at the introduction of crisaborole and tofacitinib in managing atopic dermatitis, besides age old topical steroids and calcineurin inhibitors.

Rashmi Sarkar

REFERENCES

1. Shaw T, Currie G, Koudelka C, et al. Eczema prevalence in the United States: Data from the 2003 National Survey of Children's Health. *J Invest Dermatol.* 2011;131:67-73.
2. Udkoff J, Waldman A, Ahluwalia J, et al. Current and emerging topical therapies for atopic dermatitis. *Clin Dermatol.* 2017;35:375-382.
3. Eichenfield LF, Tom WL, Berger TG, et al. Guidelines of care for the management of atopic dermatitis: Section 2. Management and treatment of atopic dermatitis with topical therapies. *J Am Acad Dermatol.* 2014;71:116-32.
4. D'Auria E, Banderali G, Barberi S, et al. Atopic dermatitis: Recent insight on pathogenesis and novel therapeutic target. *Asian Pac J Allergy Immunol.* 2016;34:98-108.
5. van Zuuren EJ, Fedorowicz Z, Christensen R, et al. Emollients and moisturisers for eczema. *Cochrane Database Syst Rev.* 2017;2:CD012119.
6. Simpson EL, Chalmers JR, Hanifin JM, et al. Emollient enhancement of the skin barrier from birth offers effective atopic dermatitis prevention. *J Allergy Clin Immunol.* 2014;134:818-23.
7. Barnes TM, Greive KA. Use of bleach baths for the treatment of infected atopic eczema. *Australas J Dermatol.* 2013;54:251-8.
8. Lee M, Van Brever H. The role of antiseptic agents in atopic dermatitis. *Asia Pac Allergy.* 2014;4:230-40.
9. Krakowski AC, Eichenfield LF, Dohil MA. Management of atopic dermatitis in the pediatric population. *Pediatrics.* 2008;122:812-24.
10. Tollefson MM, Bruckner AL. Atopic dermatitis: Skin-directed management. *Pediatrics.* 2014;134:e1735-44.

11. Simpson EL. Atopic dermatitis: A review of topical treatment options. *Curr Med Res Opin.* 2010;26:633-40.
12. Mayba JN, Gooderham MJ. Review of atopic dermatitis and topical therapies. *J Cutan Med Surg.* 2016;1-10.
13. Del Rosso J, Friedlander SF. Corticosteroids: Options in the era of steroid-sparing therapy. *J Am Acad Dermatol.* 2005;53:S50-8.
14. Chong M, Fonacier L. Treatment of eczema: corticosteroids and beyond. Clin Rev Allerg Immunol. 2016;51:249-62.
15. Katayama I, Aihara M, Ohya Y, et al. Japanese guidelines for atopic dermatitis 2017. *Allergol Int.* 2017;66:230-47.
16. Silverberg JI, Nelson DB, Yosipovitch G. Addressing treatment challenges in atopic dermatitis with novel topical therapies. *J Dermatolog Treat.* 2016;27:568-76.
17. Cury Martins J, Martins C, Aoki V, et al. Topical tacrolimus for atopic dermatitis. *Cochrane Database Syst Rev.* 2015;7:CD009864.
18. Friedlander SF, Simpson EL, Irvine AD, et al. The changing paradigm of atopic dermatitis therapy. *Semin Cutan Med Surg.* 2016;35:S97-9.
19. Siegfried EC, Jaworski JC, Kaiser JD, et al. Systematic review of published trials : Long- term safety of topical corticosteroids and topical calcineurin inhibitors in pediatric patients with atopic dermatitis. *BMC Pediatr.* 2016;16:75.
20. Gittler JK, Wang JF, Orlow SJ. Bathing and associated treatments in atopic dermatitis. *Am J Clin Dermatol.* 2017;18:45-57.
21. Dabade TS, Davis DM, Wetter DA, et al. Wet dressing therapy in conjunction with topical corticosteroids is effective for rapid control of severe pediatric atopic dermatitis: Experience with 218 patients over 30 years at Mayo Clinic. *J Am Acad Dermatol.* 2012;67:100-6.
22. Zane L, Chanda S, Jarnagin K, et al. Crisaborole and its potential role in treating atopic dermatitis: overview of early clinical studies. *Immunotherapy.* 2016;8:853-66.
23. Hoy SM. Crisaborole ointment 2%: A review in mild to moderate atopic dermatitis. *Am J Clin Dermatol.* 2017;18:837-43.
24. Damsky W, King BA. JAK inhibitors in dermatology: The promise of a new drug class. *J Am Acad Dermatol.* 2017;76:736-44.
25. Shreberk-Hassidim R, Ramot Y, Zlotogorski A. Janus kinase inhibitors in dermatology: A systematic review. *J Am Acad Dermatol.* 2017;76:745-53.
26. Bissonnette R, Papp KA, Poulin Y, et al. Topical tofacitinib for atopic dermatitis: A phase IIa randomized trial. *Br J Dermatol.* 2016;175:902-11.

World Clin Dermatol. 2018;4(1):69-80.

Treatment of Atopic Dermatitis:Systemic Therapy

[1]Paula Boggio MD, [2],*Margarita Larralde MD PhD

[1]Departments of Dermatology, Ramos Mejía Hospital and Pediatric Dermatology
Hospital Italiano de Buenos Aires, Buenos Aires, Argentina
[2]Department of Dermatology, Aleman Hospital; Department of Pediatric Dermatology
Ramos Mejía Hospital, Buenos Aires, Argentina

ABSTRACT

The majority of atopic dermatitis cases correspond to mild to moderate disease and those patients will have a satisfactory disease control with basic, topical pharmacological treatment and phototherapy. However, near one-third of cases fall into the category of moderate to severe disease, and may not achieve good control with previous measures or have a great burden of disease and a poor quality of life. For this subset of patients, systemic treatment is indicated. Current available drugs are classic immunosuppressants (cyclosporine, methotrexate, azathioprine, and mycophenolate mofetil) and the new biologic drugs which open a new era in the molecular targeted therapy of atopic dermatitis.

INTRODUCTION

The majority of atopic dermatitits (AD) patients presents mild to moderate disease that will have a satisfactory therapeutic response using appropriate emollients and avoiding irritants and triggering factors (basic treatment), together with conventional topical anti-inflammatory drugs (first-line pharmacological treatment) and/or phototherapy (second-line treatment).[1-3] Nevertheless, a subset of patients with moderate to severe disease—approximately one-third of all AD— that does not respond to topical treatment and for which phototherapy is not indicated, available or has failed, will require systemic treatment.[3,4]

*Corresponding author
Email: doctoralarralde@gmail.com

The decision of when starting a systemic immunomodulatory drug in an individual patient is complex and relies on multiple factors:[3]

- Definition of the moderate to severe AD status (considering lesional extension and severity and/or significant impact on quality of life at different time points)
- Previous optimization of topical treatment giving the patient an adequate education
- Consideration of alternative or concomitant diseases (scabies, dermatophytosis, and contact dermatitis among others)
- Indication of a trial of intensive topical therapy with posterior reevaluation of the disease burden
- Adequate treatment of infection when present
- Consideration of use of phototherapy. It is indicated for selected older children and adult patients coursing a moderate to severe disease (both acute and chronic). The most effective are narrowband ultraviolet B (NB-UVB) and ultraviolet A-1. In adults that do not respond to NB-UVB, psoralen with ultraviolet A radiation may be considered.[3,5]

DISCUSSION

When patients with moderate to severe AD do not achieve adequate control of their symptoms and signs with basic, plus first-line treatment and phototherapy, and/or the disease's clinical and psychological burden has a strong negative impact on their quality of lives, the introduction of systemic immunomodulatory drugs must be considered.[6] This group comprises nearly one-third of the adult affected population and a smaller percentage in childhood.[7]

The decision of which drug to select in a particular case should be based on patient's features (current AD status, present and past medical history, comorbidities, and personal preferences), physician's expertise, and drug availability.[5,7] In children, a careful risk/benefit analysis must be done and a main concern is the avoidance of side effects on growth or development.

The authors herein focus on main groups of drugs for AD systemic treatment.

Classic Immunomodulatory Drugs

Cyclosporine

First used in AD in 1991,[8] it is the only drug within this group approved for the Food and Drug Administration (FDA) for systemic treatment of pediatric and adult AD.[9]

Mechanism of Action

After binding to cyclophilin forms a complex that inhibits calcineurin that finally downregulates transcription of cytokines that activate T-cell, particularly interleukin (IL)-2, and also affects the balance of regulatory T-cell populations.[9]

Dosage/Regimens

Dose of 3–6 mg/kg/day in pediatric patients, 150–300 mg/day in adults, given twice a day, orally. When significant improvement is achieved and maintained, the cyclosporine should ideally be tapered or discontinued (this principle applies to all other indicated immunosuppresive drugs). Recommended time limit for continuous use is 1 year.[6,10,11] Regimens consist of starting with an initial high dose and taper after response (1 mg/kg/day every 2 weeks) until a minimum effective dose is reached; or by the contrary, start with a low dose and gradually increase it (0.5–1 mg/kg every 2 weeks) until a good response is obtained.[9]

Efficacy

Most patients have an important decrease in disease burden within 2 to 6 weeks of starting treatment.[6,10,11]

Adverse Effects

Gastrointestinal disturbances, headache, tremor and paresthesias, flu-like symptoms, hypertension, nephrotoxicity, hypertriglyceridemia, hyperkalemia, hypomagnesemia, hyperbilirubinemia, hypertrichosis, gingival hyperplasia, increased risk of infection, lymphoma, and skin cancer. Pregnancy category C.[6,10,11]

Monitoring

Baseline laboratory tests: Blood pressure measurements; renal and liver function tests, urinalysis, lipid profile, complete blood cell count, platelets, ionogram, uric acid; tuberculosis (TB) testing.[6]

Follow-up: Blood pressure at each visit; laboratory test every 2 weeks during 2–3 months, then monthly; TB testing annually. Discontinue or reduce the dose when creatinine increase greater than or equal to 30% from baseline.[6]

If clinical response is inadequate, whole-blood cyclosporine level should be determined.[6]

Special attention must be given about the interactions of cyclosporine with other systemic drugs administered simultaneously.[5]

Methotrexate

Mechanism of Action

Methotrexate (MTX) is a folic acid antagonist that inhibits the dihydrofolate reductase and blocks the synthesis of DNA, RNA, and purines, thus reducing cell proliferation.[6] It also depletes activated T-cells by an apoptosis mediated mechanism.[12] Low-dose MTX has also an immune modulator function through several mechanisms.[13]

Dosage/Regimens

Dose of 0.2–0.7 mg/kg in children and 7.5–25 mg in adults, given in a single weekly dose, oral, intramuscular, or subcutaneously. Divided total oral dose in three doses given every 12 hours is a good option when gastrointestinal intolerance is referred.[6,14] Supplementation with folic acid is highly desirable, once it reduces the likelihood of hematologic and gastrointestinal adverse effects. The recommendation is 1 mg/day, skipping the day of MTX intake.[6] Total duration of treatment varies from 4 to 38 months in different publications.[12]

Efficacy

Improvement in clinical signs and symptoms is usually seen within 6–12 weeks.[6,13] Most published case series of pediatric and adult AD patients treated with low-dose of MTX show an efficacy comparable to that of other systemic drugs for this disease. Some studies refer a slower onset of effect compared with cyclosporine, but an increased time up to relapse when discontinued.[15]

Adverse Effects

Adverse effects include nausea, vomiting and diarrhea, ulcerative stomatitis, malaise and fatigue, chills and fever, dizziness, risk of infection and malignancies, gastrointestinal ulceration and bleeding, photosensitivity, alopecia, pulmonary fibrosis and interstitial pneumonitis, elevated liver enzymes, and cytopenias. Pregnancy category X.[6,14]

Monitoring

Baseline laboratory tests: Complete blood cell count/differential/platelets, liver and renal function, hepatitis B and C serology tests, TB testing, and chest X-ray.[6,14]

Follow-up: Complete blood cell count/differential/platelets and liver function weekly during 2–4 weeks, and 1 week after each dose increase, then every 2 weeks during the first months and every 2–3 months while receiving stable doses. Renal function every 3–12 months and annual TB testing.[6,14]

Azathioprine

Mechanism of Action

Azathioprine (AZA) is a 6-mercaptopurine analog that inhibits DNA synthesis mainly affecting cells with high proliferation rates, and selectively inhibiting T lymphocytes more than B-cells during inflammatory disease states.[6] Probably it also determines a shift in the T-cell profile to a more favorable one in AD patients.[16] Its metabolization is dependent on an individual activity level of the enzyme thiopurine methyltransferase (TPMT), and drug efficacy and toxicity are related to genetic polymorphisms that determine differences in enzyme activity.[16] Therefore, baseline TPMT level testing is strongly encouraged before starting AZA treatment.[6,16]

Dosage/Regimens

Dose of 1–4 mg/kg/day in children and 1–3 mg/kg/day in adults, given orally, once a day.[6]

Efficacy

Azathioprine is effective to improve signs and symptoms of AD, as demonstrated in several trials.[17,18] Initial improvement may be seen near 6–8 weeks of treatment, but delay onset is expected, with more than or equal to 12 weeks of treatment to achieve maximum clinical benefit.[6]

Adverse Effects

Nausea, vomiting, and other gastrointestinal symptoms are common and dose related complaints. Less frequently, headache, hypersensitivity reactions, leukopenia, elevated liver enzymes, and pancreatitis are referred.[6] There is also an increased risk of developing cutaneous and lymphoproliferative malignancies with this drug. It is advisable not to use AZA simultaneously with phototherapy, because of possible photocarcinogenesis.[6,19] Pregnancy category D.[6]

Monitoring

Baseline laboratory tests: Baseline TPMT level, complete blood cell count/ differential and platelets, liver and renal function, hepatitis B and C serology tests, and TB testing.[6]

Follow-up: Complete blood cell count/differential and platelets, liver and renal function every 2 weeks during 2 months, monthly during next 4 months, and then every other month or with dose increase continuously. Annual TB testing.[6]

Mycophenolate Mofetil

Mechanism of Action

Mycophenolate mofetil (MMF) is the prodrug of mycophenolic acid (MPA)[20] that has an immunosuppressant action by blocking the *novo* purine synthesis cellular pathway through its active metabolite, MPA.[6,20,21] Specifically, it inhibits the enzyme inosine monophosphate dehydrogenase—mainly type II isoform that is predominantly located on lymphocytes, which partially explains the selective inhibition of T and B cells that MMF induces.[6,21]

Dosage/Regimen

Dose of 30–50 mg/kg/day in children (≥2 years of age), and 0.5–3 g/day for adults, administered orally twice daily.[22]

Efficacy

Mycophenolate mofetil is an effective drug in severe or refractory AD. Initial responses may be seen within the first month or delayed, and remissions seem to last longer than with cyclosporine.[6,22]

Adverse Effects

Nausea, vomiting, diarrhea, and abdominal crampingare the most frequent adverse effects (20% of patients) and are dose-dependent.[20] Rarely, hematologic compromises (anemia, leukopenia, and thrombocytopenia) and genitourinary symptoms (urgency, dysuria, hematuria, and sterile pyuria) are described. With doses of 2–3 g/day, near 20% of patients may develop fever, fatigue, back pain, acne, hypercholesterolemia, hyperglycemia, hypophosphatemia, hyper- or hypokalemia, and peripheral edema. Also, as with other immunosuppressives, a slight increased risk of infections and cutaneous tumors and lymphomas is mentioned. Pregnancy category D.[6]

Monitoring

Baseline laboratory tests: Complete blood cell count/differential and platelets, liver and renal function tests, and TB testing.[6]

Follow-up: Complete blood cell count/differential and platelets and liver and renal function tests, every 2 weeks for the first month, monthly for the next 3 months, and then every 2-3 months. Annual TB testing.[6]

Other Immunomodulatory Drugs

Interferon Gamma

Interferon gamma (IFN-γ) is a biologic response modifier with a role in both innate and adaptive immunity, that mainly enhance natural killer cell production and increase macrophage oxidation, participates in Th1 cell differentiation and also inhibits Th2 differentiation.[6,23] Few studies have demonstrated its efficacy in AD, and currently it seems particularly useful for a subset of AD patients who are deficient in IFN-γ production (those colonized with *S. aureus* and with a greater predisposition to develop eczema *herpeticum*).[23] Dosages and regimens vary, main consist of the administration of 0.5–1.5 x 10^6 UI/m², three times a week subcutaneously.[24] Primary side effects are flu-like symptoms, transaminase elevation, and transient granulocyte suppression.[5,23]

Systemic Steroids

Systemic steroids (oral or parental) should be avoided in both pediatric and adult AD patients. Although they provide a quick relief of clinical manifestations, the improvement achieved is temporary and rebound flares upon discontinuation are expected. Potential short- and long-term side effects are another discouraging point for its election. However, they could be occasionally indicated for a short period of time, while other systemic drug or phototherapy is started.[6,9]

Oral Calcineurin Inhibitors (Tacrolimus)

Oral tacrolimus has been indicated for severe AD in adults in a few studies, with variable and not encouraging results.[25] Therefore, there is still insufficient data to recommend its use.[6]

Biologic Drugs

New discoveries of the molecular pathogenic mechanisms of AD provide rationale to the various targets for treatment. It is well known at this time, that AD is mainly a Th2/Th22 inflammatory disease, but Th1 and Th17 responses modulate both the development and progression of AD.[26] Biologic drugs that have been tested for AD may be divided considering the targeted immune pathway in the following distinctive groups:[4]

Th2 Pathways Antagonists

- Dupilumab (anti-IL-4-Rα): It is a fully human monoclonal antibody targeting the shared α-subunit of IL-4 and IL-13 receptors, and therefore, the entire Th2 pathway.[4] It also induces a downregulation of Th17 and Th22 pathway genes without concomitant increases in Th1-related markers. Interleukin-4 and -13 attract T cells and eosinophils, inhibit differentiation of keratinocytes and lipid synthesis and disrupt tight junction products, promote *S. aureus* binding, and inhibit antimicrobial peptides.[4,27] Two randomized, placebo-controlled, worldwide phase III trials performed in 2016, demonstrated that dupilumab significantly improved the signs and symptoms of AD as well as the quality of life of the involved patients in a dose-dependent manner.[28] Recommended doses are 150–300 mg/week, subcutaneously. Patients reach 85% reduction of Eczema Area and Severity Index (EASI) at 12 weeks of treatment and pruritus is reduced about 55% (rating scale score) by the same time. Adverse effects are not serious, with nasopharyngitis, headache, and injection-site reactions among the most common.[29] In March 28, 2017, the FDA approved dupilumab to treat adults with moderate to severe AD
- Tralokinumab and lebrikizumab (anti-IL-13): Both are immunoglobulin G4 humanized monoclonal antibodies that bind to IL-13. Tralokinumab inhibits IL-13 binding to its receptors, a heterodimeric receptor (composed of IL4-Rα and IL-13-Rα1) and the decoy IL-13-Rα2; while lebrikizumab specifically binds soluble IL-13 at a site that overlaps with IL-4-Rα.[4] Both drugs are under clinical trials for AD and other diseases (asthma, alopecia areata, pulmonary fibrosis, and others) and seems to be well tolerated and promising in improving AD[29]
- Nemolizumab (anti-IL-31): Interleukin-31 also named the "pruritus cytokine" affects epidermal differentiation and inhibits lipid synthesis, perpetuating the "itch-scratch" cycle of AD and also seems to be implicated in disease recurrences. Nemolizumab seems to be very effective in reducing pruritis, and clinical trials are ongoing[4,29,30]
- Mepolizumab (anti-IL-5): Interleukin-5 has a critical role on biological activities of eosinophils, so the molecule itself and its receptor are the therapeutic target for hypereosinophilic diseases, in which spectrum AD is included. Mepolizumab is a fully humanized monoclonal antibody that binds to IL-5, that has been used for moderate to severe AD without relevant clinical efficacy, despite the induced decrease in peripheral blood eosinophils[31]
- Tezepelumab and OX40 ligand antagonist
- Tocilizumab (anti-IL-6).

Th22 Inhibition

- ILV-094 (anti-IL-22): Interluekin-22 is significantly upregulated in AD skin lesions (mainly in severe and chronic hyperkaratotic ones), and induces epidermal hyperplasia, inhibits epidermal differentiation, and upregulates A100 AS (together with IL17). ILV-094 is a human IgGIA antibody that binds IL-22 now under a phase IIA randomized placebo-controlled clinical trial.[4]

IgE Antagonists

Omalizumab: It is a recombinant humanized monoclonal antibody that targets the high-affinity Fc receptor of IgE, thus reducing IgE levels. Food and Drug Administration approved it for chronic urticaria and a severe allergic asthma. It has been tested in severe extrinsic AD in adults without consistent benefits.[4,32]

Th17/IL23 Antagonists

- Interleukin-23 induces Th17 and Th22, and both their products—IL-17 and 22—induce tissue inflammation and skin barrier defects. It is possible that IL-23 has also direct effects on keratinocytes, upregulating intracellular proinflammatory molecules as janus kinase 2 (JAK-2) and tyrosine kinase 2. Treatment of AD blocking this pathway might be effective in some AD subgroups (e.g., IL-17 levels are particularly high in Asian patients, in intrinsic AD, and in pediatric AD)[4]
- Ustekinumab (anti-IL-12/IL-23): Human monoclonal IgG1 against p40 subunit of IL-12 and -23. Efficacy in AD has not been significant[33]
- Secukinumab (anti-IL17): Recombinant fully human IgG1κ monoclonal antibody that selectively inhibits IL-17A. Now it is undergoing randomized, placebo-controlled trials for adult AD patients.[4]

Broader T-cell inhibition

- Apremilast: It is an oral phosphodiesterase-4 inhibitor that increase intracellular adenosine monophosphate, wich finally results in inhibition of proinflammatory cytokine production and decreased inflammation. The mechanism whereby it reduces pruritus in an independent manner of the reduction of cutaneous inflammation is not completely understood.[34] There are small case series published of adult patients with severe and refractory AD (that failed with previous topical and systemic immunosuppressive drugs), treated with apremilast 30 mg twice daily, that had noticeable improvement in burden disease within 2–4 weeks of initiating apremilast[34]

- Janus kinase (JAK) inhibitors: Janus kinase inhibitors are enzymes that phosphorylate the intracellular domain of several cytokine receptors to permit the binding and activation at the transducer and activator of transcription, that finally enters the nucleus and interfere with transcription. Janus kinase inhibitors antagonists block cytokine signaling by inhibiting down-stream of the common γc cytoplasmic receptors (shared for IL-2, -4, -9, -7, -15, and -21). Therefore, they are potent antiinflammatory and antiproliferative molecules. They can be administered orally or used topically[4,35]
- Tofacitinib (JAK 1 and 3 inhibitor): It is a pan-JAK antagonist, currently FDA approved for rheumatoid arthritis and being studied for other conditions as psoriasis and alopecia areata. It has been useful in a small case series of AD patients[36]
- Baricitinib (JAK 1 and 2 inhibitor): It is undergoing a randomized phase II placebo-controlled clinical trial for AD.[35]

CONCLUSION

Clinical management of moderate to severe AD patients is a true challenge. Regardless, well-known systemic immunomodulatory systemic drugs used up to now, the current shifting toward increased use of biologics, targeting the major immunopathogenic pathways of the disease, is very promising and a field of continuous development.

Editor's Comment

About one third of atopic dermatitis cases fall into the category of moderate-to-severe disease, and may not achieve good control with previous measures, or may have a great burden of disease and a poor quality of life. For this subset of patients systemic treatment is indicated. The article discusses the role of immunosuppressants and upcoming biologics in atopic dermatitis.

Rashmi Sarkar

REFERENCES

1. Eichenfield LF, Tom WL, Chamlin SL, et al. Guidelines of care for the management of atopic dermatitis: Section 1. Diagnosis and assesment of atopic dermatitis. *J Am Acad Dermatol.* 2014;70:338-51.
2. Bieber T. Atopic dermatitis. *Ann Dermatol.* 2010;22:125-37.
3. Simpson EL, Bruin-Weller M, Flohr C, et al. When does atopic dermatitis warrant systemic therapy? Recommendations from an expert panel of the International Eczema Council. *J Am Acad Dermatol.* 2017;77:623-33.

4. Renert-Yuval Y, Guttman-Yassky E. Systemic therapies in atopic dermatitis: The pipeline. *Clin Dermatol.* 2017;35:387-97.

5. Garritsen FM, Brouwer MW, Limpens J, et al. Photo(chemo)therapy in the management of atopic dermatitis: an updated systematic review with implications for practice and research. *Br J Dermatol.* 2014;170:501-13.

6. Sidbury R, Davis DM, Cohen DE, et al. Guidelines of care for the management of atopic dermatitis. Section 3. Management and treatment with phototherapy and systemic agents. *J Am Acad Dermatol.* 2014;71:327-49.

7. Malajian D, Guttman-Yassky E. New pathogenic and therapeutic paradigms in atopic dermatitis. *Cytokine.* 2015;73:311-18.

8. Allen B. A multicenter double-blind placebo controlled crossover to assess the efficacy and safety of cyclosporin A in adult patients with severe refractory atopic dermatitis. Athens (Greece): Royal Society of Medicine Services Ltd; 1991.

9. Slater NA, Morrell DS. Systemic therapy of childhood atopic dermatitis. *Clin Dermatol.* 2015;33:289-99.

10. Schmitt J, Schmitt N, Meurer M. Cyclosporin in the treatment of patients with atopic eczema: A systematic review and meta-analysis. *J Eur Acad Dermatol Venerol.* 2007;21:606-19.

11. Harper JI, Ahmed I, Barclay G, et al. Cyclosporin for severe childhood atopic dermatitis: short course versus continuous therapy. *Br J Dermatol.* 2000;142(1):52-8.

12. Goujon C, Berard F, Dahel K, et al. Methotrexate for the treatment of adult atopic dermatitis. *Eur J Dermatol.* 2006;16:155-8.

13. Deo M, Yung A, Hill S, et al. Methotrexate for treatment of atopic dermatitis in children and adolescents. *Int J Dermatol.* 2014;53:1037-41.

14. Kalb RE, Strober B, Weinstein G, et al. Methotrexate and psoriasis: 2009 National Psoriasis Foundation Consensus Conference. *J Am Acad Dermatol.* 2009;60:824-37.

15. El-Khalawany MA, Hassan H, Shaaban D, et al. Methotrexate versus cyclosporine in the treatment of severe atopic dermatitis in children: a multicenter experience from Egypt. *Eur J Pediatr.* 2013;172:351-56.

16. Caufield M, Tom WL. Oral azathioprine for recalcitrant pediatric atopic dermatitis: Clinical response and thiopurine monitoring. *J Am Acad Dermatol.* 2013;68:29-35.

17. Meggitt SJ, Gray JC, Reynolds NJ. Azathioprine dosed by thiopurine methyltransferase activity for moderate-to-severe atopic eczema: A double-blind, randomized controlled trial. *Lancet.* 2006;367:839-46.

18. Berth-Jones J, Takwale A, Tan E, et al. Azathioprine in severe adult atopic dermatitis: A double-blind, placebo-controlled, crossover trial. *Br J Dermatol.* 2002;147:324-30.

19. Perrett CM, Walker SL, O'Donovan P, et al. Azathioprine treatment photosensitizes human skin to ultraviolet A radiation. *Br J Dermatol.* 2008;159:198-204.

20. Orvis AK, Wesson SK, Breza TS Jr, et al. Mycophenolate mofetil in dermatology. *J Am Acad Dermatol.* 2009;60:183-99.

21. Sokumbi O, el-Azhary RA, Langman LJ. Therapeutic dose monitoring of mycophenolate mofetil in dermatologic diseases. *J Am Acad Dermatol.* 2013;68:36-40.

22. Murray ML, Cohen JB. Mycophenolate mofetil therapy for moderate to severe atopic dermatitis. *Clin Exp Dermatol.* 2007;32:23-7.

23. Brar K, Leung DY. Recent considerations in the use of recombinant interferon gamma for biological therapy for atopic dermatitis. *Expert Opin Biol Ther.* 2016;16:507-14.

24. Jang IG, Yang JK, Lee HJ, et al. Clinical improvement and immunohistochemical findings in severe atopic dermatitis treated with interferon gamma. *J Am Acad Dermatol.* 2000;42:1033-40.

25. Lee FJ, Frankum BS, Katelaris CH. Poor efficacy of oral tacrolimus in the treatment of severe generalized atopic eczema in adults: A small retrospective case series. *Australas J Dermatol.* 2012;53:295-7.

26. Kim JE, Kim JS, Cho DH, et al. Molecular mechanisms of cutaneous inflammatory disorder: Atopic dermatitis. *Int J Mol Sci.* 2016;17:1234.

27. D'erme AM, Romanelli M, Chiricozzi A. Spotlight on dupilumab in the treatment of atopic dermatitis: Design, development and potencial place in therapy. *Drug Des Devel Ther.* 2017;11:1473-80.

28. Simpson EL, Bieber T, Guttman-Yassky E, et al. Two phase 3 trials of dupilumab versus placebo in atopic dermatitis. *N Engl J Med.* 2016;375:2335-48.

29. Lauffer F, Ring J. Target-oriented therapy: emerging drugs for atopic dermatitis. *Expert Opin Emerg Drugs.* 2016;21:81-9.

30. Ruzicka T, Hanifin JM, Furue M, et al. Anti-interleukin-31 receptor A antibogy for atopic dermatitis. *N Engl J Med.* 2017;376:826-35.

31. Oldhoff JM, Darsow U, Werfel T, et al. Anti-IL-5 recombined humanized monoclonal antibody (mepolizumab) for the treatment of atopic dermatitis. *Allergy.* 2005;60:693-6.

32. Holm JG, Agner T, Sand C, et al. Omalizumab for atopic dermatitis: case series and a systematic review of the literature. *Int J Dermatol.* 2017;56:18-26.

33. Saeki H, Kabashima K, Tokura Y, et al. Efficacy and safety of ustekinumab in Japanese patients with severe atopic dermatitis: A randomized, double-blind, placebo-controlled, phase II study. *Br J Dermatol.* 2017;177:419-27.

34. Abrouk M, Farahnik B, Zhu TH, et al. Apremilast treatment of atopic dermatitis and other chronic eczematous dermatoses. *J Am Acad Dermatol.* 2017;77:177-80.

35. Damsky W, Brett KA. JAK inhibitors in dermatology: the promise of a new drug class. *J Am Acad Dermatol.* 2017;76:736-44.

36. Levy LL, Urban J, King BA. Treatment of recalcitrant atopic dermatitis with the oral Janus kinase inhibitor tofacitinib citrate. *J Am Acad Dermatol.* 2015;14:786-92.

World Clin Dermatol. 2018;4(1):81-90.

Prevention Strategies in Atopic Dermatitis

Vishal Gupta MD, Riti Bhatia MD, *Vinod K Sharma MD

Department of Dermatology and Venereology
All India Institute of Medical Sciences, New Delhi, India

ABSTRACT

"Is there something we can do to prevent eczema in our child?" is a question dermatologists often face from expectant parents, especially those with a positive history of atopy. Despite decades of exhaustive research, we still cannot claim to have a very clear answer. Recent advances in our understanding of atopic dermatitis (AD) have proposed new preventive measures. Application of emollients and dietary supplementation with probiotics seem to be promising strategies. Outlook towards certain older practices like breastfeeding and avoidance of food allergens has changed in light of newer research. Dietary supplementations, exposure to pets and avoidance of house dust mites as protective measures require further investigation. This article provides a summary of key strategies aimed at primary prevention of AD.

INTRODUCTION

In the absence of a definite cure for atopic dermatitis (AD), preventive measures assume even greater significance. As our understanding of its pathogenesis has increased, new approaches like using emollients and administration of probiotics are being evaluated as preventive strategies. New evidence regarding several age-old practices, such as infant feeding and allergen avoidance, has emerged questioning the traditional beliefs. Prevention can be at several levels—primary, secondary, or tertiary. This article deals with the strategies aimed at "primary" prevention of AD. Table 1 summarizes the various preventive strategies along with their current level of evidence.

*Corresponding author
Email: aiimsvks@yahoo.com; vksiadvl@gmail.com

Table 1: Summary of Strategies Aimed at Primary Prevention of Atopic Dermatitis and their Level of Evidence		
Intervention	Effect on atopic dermatitis	Level of evidence
Whole body emollient application	Protective	Ib
Probiotics during perinatal period	Protective	Ia
Exclusive breastfeeding for at least 3–4 months (compared to cow's milk)	No effect	IIa
Hydrolyzed milk formulas (compared to cow's milk)	Protective	Ia
Avoidance of allergenic foods in maternal diet	No effect	Ia
Maternal diet supplementation with		
• Polyunsaturated fatty acids	Protective	IIa
• Allergenic foods	Protective	IIb
• Probiotics	Protective	Ia
• Vitamin D	Not sure	IIb
Delayed introduction of allergenic foods to infant	Increases risk	IIb
Exposure to pets	Protective	IIa
Protection from house dust mite	No effect	Ia

EMOLLIENT APPLICATION BEGINNING IN EARLY LIFE

Impaired skin barrier function is now regarded as an important factor in the initiation and progression of AD. Emollients repair the skin barrier via two main mechanisms, increasing skin hydration and reducing water loss by occlusive action. By reducing the stratum corneum permeability to exogenous substances, emollients also decrease the penetration of irritants and allergens.[1] Emollients have been used regularly in the treatment of AD, and now their role in its primary prevention is also generating interest. A pilot, uncontrolled study in 2010 tested the protective effect of emollients on 22 neonates at-risk for AD (those with a first-degree relative with AD). Once-daily application of a petrolatum-based cream (Cetaphil cream, Galderma laboratories) was recommended on all body areas except scalp and diaper area. After a follow up ranging from 90 to 773 days, only 3 (15%) out of 20 children developed AD. Though comparison with historical controls suggested a protective effect, lack of a concurrent control group meant that the results could not be interpreted well. Skin barrier measurements remained within normal ranges.[2] In 2014, a randomized controlled multicentric study testing the efficacy of emollients in preventing AD in 124 high-risk neonates was published.[3] The parents in the intervention group were asked to apply emollients on full body once daily starting within 3 weeks of birth and continued until 6 months, while parents in the control group used no emollients. The various emollients offered were sunflower seed oil, Doublebase gel, liquid paraffin 50% in white soft paraffin, Cetaphil cream, and Aquaphor healing ointment. Daily emollient use reduced the cumulative incidence of AD by around 50% at 6 months (43 vs. 22%, p = 0.017). In a similar study, daily application of an emulsion-type moisturizer daily for the first 32 weeks of life was found to significantly reduce the risk of AD in high-risk neonates. Thirty-two percent (n = 19/59) in the intervention group developed AD compared to 47% (n = 28/59) in the control group (p = 0.012). However, there was no statistically significant difference in allergic sensitization to egg white between the 2 groups.[4] Though the initial results look promising, further studies on larger sample size and a longer follow-up period are required to confirm these preliminary findings. Application of emollients from neonatal period or since birth appears to be a simple, effective, and cheap method to prevent AD. A pragmatic randomized-controlled multicentric trial (the BEEP trial) involving 1,400 neonates at-risk of AD and with a longer follow-up period of 24 months is currently underway in England.[5]

ADMINISTRATION OF PROBIOTICS, PREBIOTICS, AND SYNBIOTICS IN THE PERINATAL PERIOD

Probiotics are defined as live organisms that, when administered in adequate amounts, may confer a health benefit on the host,[6] while prebiotics are indigestible carbohydrates (e.g., fructooligosaccharides, oligofructose, long-chain inulin) that promote the growth of beneficial bacterial strains in the gut.[7,8] Mixtures of probiotics and prebiotics are referred to as synbiotics. There is now good evidence to suggest the role of probiotics in preventing AD, but more data is needed to establish the role of prebiotics and synbiotics.

Most of the studies testing the efficacy of probiotics in preventing AD have employed *Lactobacillus* and *Bifidobacterium*, with *Lactobacillus rhamnosus GG* as the most frequently studied probiotic strain. Probiotics are believed to act through various mechanisms: Stimulating the Th1 cytokines while inhibiting the Th2 response thus correcting the Th1/Th2 imbalance in AD, inducing immunological tolerance by stimulating T-regulatory cells, and enhancing epithelial barrier recovery.[9] Maternal diet supplementation with probiotics can alter the immunoregulatory factors in the breast milk and may also influence the gut microbiome of the infant. A recent meta-analysis of 16 randomized placebo-controlled trials (involving 3,495 subjects) reported beneficial effect of probiotics in prevention of AD [odds ratio (OR) 0.56, 95% confidence interval (CI) 0.52–0.60, p <0.001). This protective effect was more in the high-risk group (OR 0.54, p = 0.001) compared to general population (OR 0.76, p = 0.04). Notably, probiotics exerted their effect only if administered in both prenatal as well as postnatal period. In most studies, probiotics were started 2–4 weeks before delivery and continued till 6–12 months of postnatal life. *Lactobacillus* strain, either alone or in combination with *Bifidobacterium,* was found to be protective.[10] However, two earlier studies suggested that administration of one probiotic strain may be more beneficial than combining multiple strains.[11,12] The effect of probiotic supplementation depends on multiple factors such as the probiotic strain, dose, timing and duration of administration. These factors require further investigation before probiotics can be recommended routinely for prevention of AD. On the other hand, evidence for prebiotics and synbiotics is less conclusive. A Cochrane review (4 studies, 1,218 infants) found prebiotic supplementation to reduce the risk of AD (OR 0.68, 95% CI 0.48–0.97, p = 0.03). The protective effect was more in high-risk infants compared to general population, but the difference was not statistically significant.[13] A recently published meta-analysis showed a significant effect of synbiotics in the treatment of AD (p = 0.008), but its effect in prevention was not statistically significant (OR 0.44, p = 0.26).[14]

BREASTFEEDING PRACTICES

Breastfeeding has several benefits for the infant because of its nutritional and immunological properties. It also helps in the bonding between mother and baby. The effect of exclusive breastfeeding in protecting against AD was first reported by Grulee and Sanford in 1936.[15] Since then, several studies have examined the association of breastfeeding and AD with conflicting results.[16–19]

In 2001, a meta-analysis of 18 prospective studies (involving 4,158 participants, mean follow-up period of 4.5 years) evaluating the association between breastfeeding and AD was published. Exclusive breastfeeding was shown to have a modest protective effect of 33% (OR 0.68, 95% CI 0.52–0.88) during the first 3 months of birth. This protective effect was higher for at-risk infants (OR 0.58) than in general population, while no effect was seen in infants without a family history of atopy (OR 1.43).[16] Breast milk may confer protection against AD through several mechanisms. It contains many immunomodulatory factors (IgA, cytokines, fatty acids) which help in the maturation of the infant's immune system, and helps in establishing the intestinal microflora in the infant's gut, which may polarize the immune system to Th1 response. Further, exclusive breastfeeding translates into reduced exposure to external allergens, thereby reducing the risk of sensitization. It may also protect against infections that can be a stimulus for atopy.[16,17] A Cochrane review showed that hydrolyzed milk formula and breast milk had a similar effect in preventing AD.[20] The protection by hydrolyzed milk is directly proportional to the degree of hydrolysis.[21] Supplementing breast milk with formula feeds after the initial 3 months does not appear to reduce its protective effect, with some studies suggesting no additional advantage of extending exclusive breast feeding to 6 months.[22-24] In 2008, the American Academy of Pediatrics (AAP) stated that exclusive breastfeeding for at-least 4 months or breast milk supplemented with hydrolyzed formula (compared to supplementation with cow milk-based formula) decreases the risk of AD in infants at-risk of atopy.[25] However, this statement has been questioned in light of recent studies showing no or even a positive association between breastfeeding and AD.[29]

In an observational prospective study following a cohort of 1,314 infants for 7 years, the risk of AD was shown to increase with each additional month of breastfeeding. However, the authors noted positive family history to be a confounding factor; infants with a family history of eczema were more likely to be breastfed for a longer period (reverse causation).[27] Another prospective cohort study from Japan involving 763 infants showed no overall risk of AD in breastfed infants during the first 16–24 months of life. However, the authors found breastfeeding to be a risk factor for AD in children with a negative family history of allergic diseases.[28] A cross-sectional study on 10,383 Korean children aged 0–13 years reported prolonged breastfeeding (>12 months) as a risk factor for AD in children <5 years of age (but not in those >5 years), regardless of family history of atopy.[29] Another meta-analysis of 21 prospective cohort studies (34,227 participants, with a mean follow-up duration of 2.2 years), with significant heterogeneity across the studies, reported only a mild overall reduction in AD in breastfed children (OR 0.89, 95% CI 0.76–1.04). Exclusive breastfeeding was found to be more protective when compared to formula feeding (OR 0.70) as against partial breastfeeding (OR 0.95). The protective effect was slightly more in children with a positive family history of atopy (OR 0.78, 95% CI 0.58–1.05) than in those with a negative family history (OR 0.93, 95% CI 0.60–1.45) but the difference was not statistically significant. Interestingly, the more recent was the publication the less was the protective effect of breastfeeding, probably because of adjustment for confounders in the newer studies. Further, the effect was seen to decrease with increasing follow-up duration suggesting that exclusive breastfeeding only delays the onset of AD and does not prevent it altogether.[17] The final word on the effect of breastfeeding on AD is not out yet. Studies conducted so far have several limitations such as recall bias, limited follow-up period, self-reporting of AD, and potential confounding factors including reverse causation. The atopic status of the mother appears to influence the effect of breastfeeding, and also requires further investigation.

CHANGES IN MATERNAL DIET DURING PREGNANCY/LACTATION

In 2000, the AAP stated that exclusive breastfeeding has a protective effect against AD, particularly when combined with maternal avoidance of cow's milk, egg, fish, peanuts, and tree nuts during lactation.[30] This recommendation was based on previous studies, however, several confounding factors like length of breastfeeding, use of supplemental feeds, and introduction of solid foods to infants were not controlled for in many trials. Two Cochrane reviews (four randomized controlled trials, 334 participants)[31] and (5 trials, 952 participants)[32] found no effect of maternal dietary antigen avoidance during pregnancy on the incidence of AD during the first 18 months of life. On the contrary, it may be associated with a lower maternal weight gain, prematurity, and low birth weight. Similarly, maternal antigen avoidance during lactation was also found to have no significant protective effect.[32] Lack of protective effect in many studies could also be attributed to "reverse causation," as the parents of children with AD are more likely to adhere to dietary allergen avoidance.

Now, the focus is shifting from food avoidance towards maternal diet supplementation. There is preliminary evidence that dietary intake of common food allergens by the mother during pregnancy may, in fact, have a protective role. A prospective cohort study on 1,277 subjects found higher maternal wheat intake during the second trimester reduced the risk of AD in mid-childhood (OR 0.64, 95% CI 0.46–0.90).[33] Another similar study on 1,354 mother-child pairs from Japan reported reduced risk of infantile eczema with higher maternal intake of dairy products (OR 0.64), yogurt (OR 0.49), and calcium (OR 0.34), while maternal intake of vitamin D was associated with a higher risk of infantile eczema (OR 1.63).[34] Interestingly, in a prospective study on 763 participants, the same authors had earlier reported maternal vitamin D intake (>4.309 µg/day) to be associated with reduced risk (OR 0.63) of childhood eczema in infants aged 16–24 months.[35] The 2016 World Allergy Organization guidelines suggest against vitamin D supplementation for preventing allergic diseases, while acknowledging that this recommendation is based on currently available low-quality evidence.[36] A meta-analysis of 13 studies evaluating the role of maternal dietary supplementation with omega-3-long chain polyunsaturated fatty acids during pregnancy in preventing allergic diseases showed a significant reduction in AD (OR 0.53, 95% CI 0.35–0.81). However, due to the inconsistency of results, the effect of maternal polyunsaturated fatty acids could not be confirmed beyond doubt.[37] The effect of probiotic supplementation in the maternal diet has been discussed earlier.

EARLY INTRODUCTION OF ALLERGENIC FOODS TO INFANTS

Studies suggest that there may be a critical period in infancy when a child inherently predisposed to allergic diseases is at a higher risk of being sensitized. It was earlier believed that early introduction of allergenic foods would increase the risk of allergic diseases, because of the immature immune system and increased gut permeability in early infancy.[38] The common food allergens during childhood include cow's milk, hen's egg, soy, wheat, peanut, tree nuts, and fish. In 2000, the AAP recommended delaying the introduction of certain allergenic foods.[30] These recommendations were based more on consensus than direct evidence. Later, studies were published which suggested that delayed introduction of certain foods such as wheat and peanuts, in fact, increased the risk of allergy to that specific food.[39,40] A Dutch prospective birth cohort study on 2,558 infants found introduction of cow's milk after 7 months of age to be associated with a higher risk of eczema at 2 years of age.[41] In light of these newer studies, the AAP changed its stance in 2008—avoidance of any allergenic food beyond 4–6 months of age was no longer recommended.[25] Most of the current evidence on early introduction of allergenic foods deals with risk of food allergy and sensitization. More studies are needed to confirm if this protective effect can be extrapolated to AD as well.

EXPOSURE TO HOUSE PETS

As per the hygiene hypothesis, reduced exposure to microbes and other infectious agents in early life can have an impact on the maturation of the immune system, predisposing the children to allergic and autoimmune diseases. Regular contact with animals may be associated with reduced risk of atopy and other allergic diseases. A recent meta-analysis of 21 birth cohort studies reported a 25% reduction in the risk of AD in children exposed to pets (OR 0.75, 95% CI 0.67–0.85), particularly dogs (OR 0.72, 95% CI 0.61–0.85). Exposure to cats was not found to have a significant effect (OR 0.94, 95% CI 0.76–1.16). The authors suggested that the difference in the skin and mucosal microbiomes between dogs and cats may explain their differing effects on AD.[42]

PROTECTION FROM HOUSE DUST MITES

The role of house dust mite in causing AD is debatable.[43] Despite lack of evidence, dust mite avoidance is commonly recommended in treatment as well as prevention of AD. Some studies have shown that decreasing the levels of dust mite allergen may have no significant effect on reducing AD or sensitisation.[44-46] A meta-analysis of 3 randomized controlled trials examining the effect of preventing house dust mite exposure in at-risk infants did not find any significant effect (OR 1.08, 95% CI 0.78–1.49) in preventing AD.[47] Protection from house dust mite was observed by using mite impermeable mattress encasings for infants and parents and/or acaricidal treatments, while the control group used standard cotton mattresses. The studies included in the meta-analysis had inconsistent methodology and were done on a small sample size. Until better randomized controlled trials are conducted, avoidance of house dust mite allergen cannot be recommended as a preventive measure.

CONCLUSION

Systematic reviews and meta-analysis have been conducted with the aim to provide a clear answer regarding the protective role of individual measures, however, evidence is still not enough to reach a definite conclusion. It is unlikely that a single measure would protect against a disease as complex as AD. So far, most of the studies have targeted the at-risk population. However, this approach has been questioned as it would miss out on a substantial proportion of patients who develop AD in the absence of these risk factors. The recent advances in the pathogenesis of AD have prompted re-evaluation of many traditional preventive strategies. New ideas need to be tested carefully in a scientifically correct manner so that these can stand the test of time.

Editor's Comment

A part of general measures in atopic dermatitis is delineating preventive strategies to the parents. Application of emollients and dietary supplementation with probiotics seem to be promising strategies. Certain older practices like breastfeeding and avoidance of food allergens has changed in light of newer research. Dietary supplementations, exposure to pets, and avoidance of house dust mites as protective measures require further investigations.

Rashmi Sarkar

REFERENCES

1. Wirén K, Nohlgård C, Nyberg F, et al. Treatment with a barrier-strengthening moisturizing cream delays relapse of atopic dermatitis: A prospective and randomized controlled clinical trial. *J Eur Acad Dermatol Venereol*. 2009;23:1267-72.
2. Simpson EL, Berry TM, Brown PA, et al. A pilot study of emollient therapy for the primary prevention of atopic dermatitis. *J Am Acad Dermatol*. 2010;63:587-93.
3. Simpson EL, Chalmers JR, Hanifin JM, et al. Emollient enhancement of the skin barrier from birth offers effective atopic dermatitis prevention. *J Allergy Clin Immunol*. 2014;134:818-23.
4. Horimukai K, Morita K, Narita M, et al. Application of moisturizer to neonates prevents development of atopic dermatitis. *J Allergy Clin Immunol*. 2014;134:824-30.e6.
5. Chalmers JR, Haines RH, Mitchell EJ, et al. Effectiveness and cost-effectiveness of daily all-over-body application of emollient during the first year of life for preventing atopic eczema in high-risk children (The BEEP trial): Protocol for a randomised controlled trial. *Trials*. 2017;18:343.
6. Hill C, Guarner F, Reid G, et al. Expert consensus document. The International Scientific Association for Probiotics and Prebiotics consensus statement on the scope and appropriate use of the term probiotic. *Nat Rev Gastroenterol Hepatol*. 2014;11:506-14.
7. Gibson GR, Roberfroid MB. Dietary modulation of the human colonic microbiota: introducing the concept of prebiotics. *J Nutr*. 1995;125:1401-12.

8. Collins MD, Gibson GR. Probiotics, prebiotics, and synbiotics: Approaches for modulating the microbial ecology of the gut. *Am J Clin Nutr*. 1999;69:1052S-57S.

9. Rather IA, Bajpai VK, Kumar S, et al. Probiotics and atopic dermatitis: An overview. *Front Microbiol*. 2016;7:507.

10. Panduru M, Panduru NM, Sălăvăstru CM, et al. Probiotics and primary prevention of atopic dermatitis: A meta-analysis of randomized controlled studies. *J Eur Acad Dermatol Venereol*. 2015;29:232-42.

11. Doege K, Grajecki D, Zyriax B-C, et al. Impact of maternal supplementation with probiotics during pregnancy on atopic eczema in childhood--a meta-analysis. *Br J Nutr*. 2012;107:1-6.

12. Pelucchi C, Chatenoud L, Turati F, et al. Probiotics supplementation during pregnancy or infancy for the prevention of atopic dermatitis: A meta-analysis. *Epidemiol Camb Mass*. 2012;23:402-14.

13. Osborn DA, Sinn JK. Prebiotics in infants for prevention of allergy. *Cochrane Database Syst Rev*. 2013;CD006474.

14. Chang Y-S, Trivedi MK, Jha A, et al. Synbiotics for prevention and treatment of atopic dermatitis: A meta-analysis of randomized clinical trials. *JAMA Pediatr*. 2016;70:236-42.

15. Grulee CG, Sanford HN. The influence of breast and artificial feeding on infantile eczema. *J Pediatr*. 1936;9:223-5.

16. Gdalevich M, Mimouni D, David M, et al. Breast-feeding and the onset of atopic dermatitis in childhood: A systematic review and meta-analysis of prospective studies. *J Am Acad Dermatol*. 2001;45:520-7.

17. Yang YW, Tsai CL, Lu CY. Exclusive breastfeeding and incident atopic dermatitis in childhood: A systematic review and meta-analysis of prospective cohort studies. *Br J Dermatol*. 2009;161:373-83.

18. Dattner AM. Breastfeeding and atopic dermatitis: protective or harmful? facts and controversies. *Clin Dermatol*. 2010;28:34-7.

19. Kim JH. Role of breast-feeding in the development of atopic dermatitis in early childhood. *Allergy Asthma Immunol Res*. 2017;9:285-7.

20. Osborn DA, Sinn J. Formulas containing hydrolysed protein for prevention of allergy and food intolerance in infants. *Cochrane Database Syst Rev*. 2006;CD003664.

21. de Boissieu D. Do breast-feeding and "diet" milks have any preventive or curative effect in the management of atopic dermatitis in children? *Ann Dermatol Venereol*. 2005;132 Spec No 1:1S104-111.

22. Laubereau B, Brockow I, Zirngibl A, et al. Effect of breast-feeding on the development of atopic dermatitis during the first 3 years of life—results from the GINI-birth cohort study. *J Pediatr*. 2004;144:602-7.

23. Schoetzau A, Filipiak-Pittroff B, Franke K, et al. Effect of exclusive breast-feeding and early solid food avoidance on the incidence of atopic dermatitis in high-risk infants at 1 year of age. *Pediatr Allergy Immunol*. 2002;13:234-42.

24. von Berg A, Koletzko S, Grübl A, et al. German Infant Nutritional Intervention Study Group. The effect of hydrolyzed cow's milk formula for allergy prevention in the first year of life: The German Infant Nutritional Intervention Study, a randomized double-blind trial. *J Allergy Clin Immunol*. 2003;111:533-40.

25. Greer FR, Sicherer SH, Burks AW, et al. Effects of early nutritional interventions on the development of atopic disease in infants and children: The role of maternal dietary restriction, breastfeeding, timing of introduction of complementary foods, and hydrolyzed formulas. *Pediatrics*. 2008;121:183-91.

26. Risch AC. Breastfeeding and atopic dermatitis. Pediatrics. 2012;130:e461-462; author reply e465-466.

27. Bergmann RL, Diepgen TL, Kuss O, et al. Breastfeeding duration is a risk factor for atopic eczema. *Clin Exp Allergy*. 2002;32:205-9.

28. Miyake Y, Tanaka K, Sasaki S, et al. Breastfeeding and atopic eczema in Japanese infants: The Osaka Maternal and Child Health Study. *Pediatr Allergy Immunol*. 2009;20:234-41.

29. Hong S, Choi W-J, Kwon H-J, et al. Effect of prolonged breast-feeding on risk of atopic dermatitis in early childhood. *Allergy Asthma Proc*. 2014;35:66-70.

30. American Academy of Pediatrics. Committee on Nutrition. Hypoallergenic infant formulas. *Pediatrics*. 2000; 106:346-9.

31. Kramer MS, Kakuma R. Maternal dietary antigen avoidance during pregnancy or lactation, or both, for preventing or treating atopic disease in the child. *Cochrane Database Syst Rev*. 2006;CD000133.

32. Kramer MS, Kakuma R. Maternal dietary antigen avoidance during pregnancy or lactation, or both, for preventing or treating atopic disease in the child. *Cochrane Database Syst Rev.* 2012;CD000133.

33. Bunyavanich S, Rifas-Shiman SL, Platts-Mills TA, et al. Peanut, milk, and wheat intake during pregnancy is associated with reduced allergy and asthma in children. *J Allergy Clin Immunol.* 2014;133:1373-82.

34. Miyake Y, Tanaka K, Okubo H, et al. Maternal consumption of dairy products, calcium, and vitamin D during pregnancy and infantile allergic disorders. *Ann Allergy Asthma Immunol.* 2014;113:82-7.

35. Miyake Y, Sasaki S, Tanaka K, et al. Dairy food, calcium and vitamin D intake in pregnancy, and wheeze and eczema in infants. *Eur Respir J.* 2010;35:1228-34.

36. Yepes-Nuñez JJ, Fiocchi A, Pawankar R, et al. World Allergy Organization-McMaster University Guidelines for Allergic Disease Prevention (GLAD-P): Vitamin D. *World Allergy Organ J.* 2016;9:17.

37. Best KP, Gold M, Kennedy D, et al. Omega-3 long-chain PUFA intake during pregnancy and allergic disease outcomes in the offspring: A systematic review and meta-analysis of observational studies and randomized controlled trials. *Am J Clin Nutr.* 2016;103:128-43.

38. Høst A, Koletzko B, Dreborg S, et al. Dietary products used in infants for treatment and prevention of food allergy. Joint Statement of the European Society for Paediatric Allergology and Clinical Immunology (ESPACI) Committee on Hypoallergenic Formulas and the European Society for Paediatric Gastroenterology, Hepatology and Nutrition (ESPGHAN) Committee on Nutrition. *Arch Dis Child.* 1999;81:80-4.

39. Poole JA, Barriga K, Leung DY, et al. Timing of initial exposure to cereal grains and the risk of wheat allergy. *Pediatrics.* 2006;117:2175-82.

40. Du Toit G, Katz Y, Sasieni P, et al. Early consumption of peanuts in infancy is associated with a low prevalence of peanut allergy. *J Allergy Clin Immunol.* 2008;122:984-91.

41. Snijders BE, Thijs C, van Ree R, et al. Age at first introduction of cow milk products and other food products in relation to infant atopic manifestations in the first 2 years of life: The KOALA Birth Cohort Study. *Pediatrics.* 2008;122:e115-122.

42. Pelucchi C, Galeone C, Bach J-F, et al. Pet exposure and risk of atopic dermatitis at the pediatric age: A meta-analysis of birth cohort studies. *J Allergy Clin Immunol.* 2013;132:616-622.e7.

43. Fuiano N, Incorvaia C. Dissecting the causes of atopic dermatitis in children: Less foods, more mites. *Allergol Int.* 2012;61:231-43.

44. Marks GB, Mihrshahi S, Kemp AS, et al. Prevention of asthma during the first 5 years of life: A randomized controlled trial. *J Allergy Clin Immunol.* 2006;118:53-61.

45. Woodcock A, Lowe LA, Murray CS, et al. Early life environmental control: effect on symptoms, sensitization, and lung function at age 3 years. *Am J Respir Crit Care Med.* 2004;170:433-9.

46. Schönberger HJ, Dompeling E, Knottnerus JA, et al. The PREVASC study: The clinical effect of a multifaceted educational intervention to prevent childhood asthma. *Eur Respir J.* 2005;25:660-70.

47. Bremmer SF, Simpson EL. Dust mite avoidance for the primary prevention of atopic dermatitis: A systematic review and meta-analysis. *Pediatr Allergy Immunol.* 2015;26:646-54.

World Clin Dermatol. 2018;4(1):91-9.

Allergens and Atopic Dermatitis

[1,]*Sandipan Dhar MBBS DNB DVD FRGUHS
[2]Sahana M Srinivas MBBS DNB DVD FRGUHS

[1]Department of Pediatric Dermatology, Institute of Child Health
Kolkata, West Bengal, India
[2]Department of Pediatric Dermatology, Indira Gandhi Institute of Child Health
Bangalore, Karnataka, India

ABSTRACT

Atopic dermatitis is a chronic itchy inflammatory skin disease which starts early in life. The role of allergen and atopic dermatitis is complex. Allergic sensitization is seen in children probably due to primary barrier defect and inflammatory eczema. The variation in presentation of atopic dermatitis in different regions is related to gene environment interactions and the environmental factors that influence skin barrier function. Various allergens that have shown risk factor in atopic dermatitis include aeroallergens, pollution, food allergens, and irritants like wool, nickel, microbial exposure, and topical contact sensitizers. This article reviews the various allergens associated with the atopic dermatitis risk and their pathophysiology in association with atopic dermatitis.

INTRODUCTION

Atopic dermatitis (AD) is a chronic, relapsing, pruritic, inherited inflammatory skin disorder that begins in infancy or early childhood. Atopic dermatitis is a result of complex interplay of environmental, food, drugs, allergens, and immunological factors in genetically predisposed individuals.[1] Immune responses in AD occur through the skin in response to various allergens. The quality of immune responses to the allergens depends on the skin barrier, the type of antigen, and the cellular networks present in the skin at the time of allergen contact.[2,3] There is induction of specific Th2 cells and increase in serum immunoglobulin E (IgE) levels in

---

*Corresponding author
Email: doctorsandipan@gmail.com

Table 1: Various Allergens Associated with Atopic Dermatitis

- Environmental—Pollution, tobacco smoke, volatile organic compounds
- Aeroallergens—Dust mites, pollens, animal dander, mold
- Food allergens—Milk, milk products, egg, wheat, soy, peanuts, seafood, shellfish
- Irritants—Nickel, latex, wood, chemicals like soap, formaldehyde, balsam of Peru, dinitrochlorobenzene, sodium lauryl sulfate
- Microbial allergens—Bacterial allergens, helminth parasites, viruses (human herpes virus), fungi (*Malasezzia*)
- Clothing—Wool, synthetic fibers
- Medication allergens—Moisturizers, skin care products (fragrance), preservatives, propylene glycol, cocamidopropyl betaine, lanolin, antibiotics, corticosteroids

response to allergens. There is lot of debate over the last few years regarding the exact role of allergens in AD, leading to immune dysregulation. Allergens involved in AD are mainly exogenous factors. Factors involved are environmental triggers, aeroallergens like pollens, house dust mite (HDM), pet dander, fungi, molds, food allergens, drugs, insect venoms, and contact sensitization (Table 1).[4] Various allergens and their pathophysiology in association with AD are discussed in this article.

ALLERGENS AND SKIN BARRIER FUNCTION

Many studies in the past have overemphasized about the role of allergy in AD. Although there is an allergic sensitization in AD, the main mechanism is due to primary barrier defect and inflammatory eczema.[5] Inflamed skin and defective barrier in AD leads to penetration of allergens that further triggers the immune response and IgE mediated allergens. There is strong evidence that genetic factors and environmental triggers play an important role in predisposition of AD. Though there are over 80 candidate gene, role of barrier dysfunction genes is mainly targeted. Gene encoding filaggrin (*FLG*) has been associated as a risk factor for development of AD. Loss of function mutation in the *FLG* gene results in barrier dysfunction. Environmental factors precipitate the polygenic risk background to disease manifestation.[6] Prevailing evidence has shown that allergen sensitization is not a cause of AD, but it is probably due to consequence of AD and exogenous factors plays an important role in aggravating AD. *Filaggrin* gene mutation is also associated as a risk factor for development of 'atopic march'. Atopic march is the tendency of AD to develop into food allergies, asthma and allergic rhinitis in a temporal sequence.[7-9] *Filaggrin* defects were correlated with disease severity and allergen response. Infants with increase in transepidermal water loss (TEWL) at

2 days of life have shown increased IgE positivity to food at 2 years of age even in the absence of clinical features of AD.[10]

ALLERGEN AND IMMUNEDYSREGULATION

Immune dysregulation was the key to the pathogenesis of AD, but recently skin barrier defects play an important role in causation of AD. There is impairment of both adaptive and innate immunity in children with AD. In AD there is a dysbalance between Th1 and Th2 response with predominance of Th2 response especially in acute phase. There is increased expression of IgE receptors on Langerhans cell and dendritic cells in epidermis that present antigen to adaptive immune system. There is increase in expression of interleukin (IL)-4 and IL-33, thymic stromal lymphoprotein (TSLP) in epidermis associated with Th2 inflammation.[3,11] Thymic stromal lymphoprotein also exerts its effect on mast cells, basophils, and eosinophils involved in inflammation. Intrinsic enzymatic activity and exogenous protease activity of allergens disrupts the epidermal tight junction and induces inflammatory mediators IL-6, IL-8, and granulocyte-macrophage colony-stimulating factor from keratinocytes.[12] Protease activated receptor-2 expressed in keratinocytes is enhanced by ultraviolet rays which may explain the seasonal variation seen in AD and development of AD.[13]

ALLERGENS IN ATOPIC DERMATITIS

Environmental Allergens

Numerous factors from the environment have been thought to be associated with aggravation of AD. Air pollution, volatile organic compounds, and traffic exhaust in outdoor have been associated with development of maintenance of AD. There are studies documenting the evidence for exposure to certain factors causing switch towards AD in early life. Questionnaire based studies from Sweden and East Germany regarding the association of between outdoor pollution and atopic dermatitis has shown increased risk in individuals living close to heavy traffic.[14] However, similar studies from East Germany, Russia, and Japan did not confirm this finding.[15] Many cohort studies and cross-section survey in children have shown that fine particle pollutants (NO_2 exposure) have increased risk of AD.[16-18] There are studies of similar positive association with outdoor pollution in rural setting also.[19] There is lack of evidence regarding the association of maternal smoking during pregnancy or environmental exposure postnatally with risk of AD in offspring. Exposure to environmental tobacco smoke was associated with significant risk of developing AD especially in children with atopic background.[20]

Aeroallergens

Aeroallergens are most frequently associated with atopic diathesis. Among the aeroallergens, the most common allergen is HDMs. House dust mites belong to the species *Dermatophagoides pteronyssinus* and *Dermatophagoides farina*. House dust mite accompany humans and present in dust from mattress or bedroom floors. Some researches claim that HDM allergy is just an epiphenomenon as a result of impaired skin barrier and they do not have a direct causative role in AD.[21] Encasings of mattress and beddings give protection from mites contained in mattresses, but few randomized controlled trials did not show this effect. Mite proof pajamas are also available which improve AD. Many studies have shown improvement of AD with HDM avoidance strategies.[22]

Ragweed pollens in outdoor especially in spring and summer time can exacerbate atopic dermatitis and this has been documented in nested case control study in preschool children.[23] As complete avoidance of pollen in outdoor is practically impossible, air conditioning with pollen filters used indoors may improve AD.

Animal dander and pet exposure has shown to deteriorate symptoms of AD. Direct contact with farm animals reduces the risk of AD in early life in few studies.[24] This protective effect is more during pregnancy and even stronger in who are exposed pre- and postnatally. Cat epithelia exposure is a risk factor for exacerbation of AD. A meta-analysis of studies has shown uniform protective effect of dog exposure but not to cat.[25] Cat sensitization has been associated with *FLG* mutation inheritance with impaired skin barrier, contributing risk factor for AD.[26] Consumption of unpasteurized milk during the first 2 years of life has protective effect against AD. Once the raw milk is boiled the protective effect is lost. The mechanism of this protective effect is exactly not known and possibly attributed to the microbial contamination.[27] Risk reduction in AD seen with farm animals and pet exposure in pregnancy probably is related to high endotoxin exposure, a group of lipopolysaccharides found on the surface of gram-negative bacteria and is known to induce IL-10 and interferon-γ. Birth cohort studies have shown 50% reduction in AD with high endotoxin exposure.[28] Allergen specific immunotherapy has been found to be useful in treating aeroallergens triggered AD.

Irritants

Irritant reactions to chemicals and metals exacerbate AD (Table 1). Soaps can act as irritant in AD, thereby increasing the dryness and TEWL. Alkaline nature of the soap can increase the pH of skin altering the skin barrier. Recently, it has been shown that removal of such irritants or avoidance from birth can reduce AD.[29]

Hardness of water could act as an irritant and increase AD, but recently studies from Spain have questioned about the validity of previous studies. Increased skin pH of skin downregulates the expression and exacerbate AD. Early ear piercing and use of nickel releasing jewelry has been associated with increased nickel contact allergy in AD. Nickel contact allergy has been associated with *FLG* gene deficiency. Nickel which is electrophilic in nature binds to FLG metabolite cis-urocanic acid in human skin. Allergic contact dermatitis to nickel has been reported in younger age group with FLG mutation carriers and showed positive patch test reactivity than those without mutations.[30]

Though experimental studies have shown significant reduced risk of contact sensitization (CS) in AD, few studies have shown that the percutaneous penetration of both lipophilic and hydrophilic chemicals was increased in clinically normal skin in AD than healthy subjects and this significantly correlated with increasing severity and total serum IgE.[31] One study has shown CS to dinitrochlorobenzene in AD individuals with 100% reactivity in mild disease, 95% in moderate and 35% with severe disease.[32] However, this inverse relationship is still debated and controversial. Latex allergy in atopic dermatitis with positive patch test has shown strong Th2 response. This could be explained as AD patients with lower degree of sensitization have a stewing towards Th2 response than Th1 response. Patients with AD have been associated with increased diffusion to both polyethylene glycols and sodium lauryl sulfate as compared to normal subjects.[33]

Drug Allergens

Contact sensitization to topical allergens is well documented in AD. Contact allergy can occur to moisturizers, topical steroids, and calcineurin inhibitors which are widely used in AD. In a recent study, it has shown that these products contain one or more potent allergens (fragrances, preservatives, propylene glycol) that can exacerbate AD.[34] There is increased prevalence of CS to corticosteroids, tixocortol pivalate, and chlorhexidine. This association of CS to topical products was strongly associated with FLG mutation.[35] Use of over the counter topical medications and personal skin care products containing cocamidopropyl betaine and lanolin were known to exacerbate AD. Several studies have shown higher prevalence of CS to fragrance in AD, but few studies have disapproved an association.[36] There is a casual link between antibiotics and increased risk of developing AD. Longitudinal studies have shown overall risk increased by 41% in those who received antibiotics in early life. This increased risk is possibly due to changes in host microbiome and altered immune responses to environmental allergens.[37] There is no evidence that routine childhood vaccinations influence AD risk.

Clothes and Textile Allergy

Coarse fabrics like woolen and synthetic clothes exacerbate AD. Smooth clothing, preferably cotton clothes, and avoidance of irritating fabrics is necessary to prevent exacerbation of AD.[38]

Microbial Allergens

Microbial exposure influences the development of AD either by triggering or aggravating AD. There is altered skin microbiome in AD. These microbial pathogens induce host production of superantigen or pathogen specific IgE leasing to mast cell degranulation and Th2 mediated response. Children with AD are prone to skin infections with *Staphylococcal aureus*.[39] Both lesional and nonlesional skin in AD is colonized with *S. aureus* that acts as a trigger for skin symptoms. There is increased proinflammatory cytokines (IL-4, IL-13, TSLP), thus enhancing skin barrier disruption and penetration of environmental allergens.[40] *Staphylococcus aureus* produces enterotoxin that induces enterotoxin specific IgE resulting in proliferation and recruitment of more T cells and aggravation of AD.[41] Sensitization to *Malassezia* seen specifically in AD manifests on face and neck. Prick test and *Malassezia*-specific IgE may be positive and has a tendency towards Th2 immune response.[42] Cutaneous viral infections like warts, human herpes virus, molluscum contagiosum are more prevalent and resistant in AD. Atopic dermatitis patients are prone to eczema herpeticum and recently have been shown to be associated with FLG mutation. There is no evidence of increased risk of dermatophyte infections in AD.[29] Double blind randomized controlled trial with deworming therapy conducted among more than 2,500 pregnant mothers in a helminth endemic area in Uganda in the last trimester found two times increased AD risk up to 1 year of age. Priming of immune system in perinatal period can provide protection against AD.[43] There is conflicting reports of influence of perinatal infections on AD in the offspring.

Food Allergens

Role of diet in development and exacerbation of AD is controversial and not well defined.[44] Studies have shown the prevalence of food allergy in AD from 20 to 80%. Prevalence of food allergy proven by double blind placebo controlled studies (DBPCFC) was 33–63%. Common food allergens known to trigger AD are milk and milk products, peanuts, egg, soy, wheat, seafood, and shellfish. An open pilot study conducted by Dhar et al. on the effects of dietary elimination in AD in 100 Indian children showed statistically significant decrease in the severity score after dietary elimination alone.[45] On the contrary, few studies have not shown any association of food allergy and AD. There is increased binding of antigen to immature gut microvillus, increased intestinal permeability that initiates immune responses, with primarily altered antigen transfer. The gut bacterial pathogen acts as infectious agent and super antigen, thus exacerbating AD by food.[44] Food allergy manifests as early or late reactions. Immediate IgE mediated reactions occurs within few minutes to hours after ingestion of food allergen. Clinically presents as urticaria, angioedema, pruritus, erythema, contact urticaria, morbilliform eruptions, and allergic contact dermatitis. Late reactions can occur after 2–6 days. Cochrane systemic review based on randomized controlled trials have shown that dietary elimination did not show any improvement in AD.[46] Many patients may have sensitization to food but without clinical symptoms. Sensitization to food can be confirmed by increased serum IgE, skin prick test, skin application food test, radioallergensorbent test, atopic patch test, and oral challenge test (DBPCFC). In an Indian study by Dhar et al, skin prick test positivity to common food allergens were egg white, fish, milk, brinjal, dal, groundnut, and banana.[47] The DBPCFC is the gold standard for diagnosing food allergy. Elimination diet should be followed only if proven food allergy is present.

CONCLUSION

Allergens play an important role in the pathogenesis of AD. Atopic dermatitis is a complex interplay between impaired skin barrier and multiple allergens causing dysfunction immune response. *Filaggrin* gene mutation predisposes these allergens to trigger or aggravate AD. Understanding these factors and counseling patients of avoidance strategies can prevent aggravation of AD.

Editor's Comment

Various allergens that have shown risk factors in atopic dermatitis include aeroallergens, pollution, food allergens, and irritants like wool, nickel, microbial exposure and topical contact sensitizers. Filaggrin gene mutation predisposes these allergens to trigger or aggravate AD. The avoidance and prevention of these allergic agents is an important strategy in managing atopic dermatitis.

Rashmi Sarkar

REFERENCES

1. Dhar S, Banerjee R. Atopic dermatitis in infants and children in India. *Indian J Dermatol Venereol Leprol.* 2010;16:504-13.
2. Dhar S. Current concepts about the management of atopic dermatitis in infants and children. *Ann Inst Child Health.* 2004;4:19-28.
3. Smith AR, Knaysi G, Wilson JM, et al. The skin as a route of allergen exposure: Part 1. Immune components and mechanism. *Curr Allergt Asthma Rep.* 2017;17:6.
4. Knaysi G, Smith AR, Wilson JM, et al. The skin as a route of allergen exposure: Part II. Allergens and role of microbiome and environmental exposure. *Curr Allergy Asthma Rep.* 2017;17:7.
5. Flohr C, Weiland SK, Weinmayr G, et al. The role of atopic sensitization in flexural eczema: Findings from the international study of asthma and allergies in childhood phase two. *J Allergy Clin Immunol.* 2008;121:141-7.
6. Boguniewicz M, Leung DY. Atopic dermatitis: A disease of altered skin barrier and immune dysregulation. *Immunol Rev.* 2011;242:233-46.
7. Hahn EL, Bacharier LB. The atopic march: The pattern of allergic disease development in childhood. *Immunol Allergy Clin North Am.* 2005;25:231-46.
8. Dhar S, Kanwar AJ, Nagraja. Personal and family history of 'atopy' in children with atopic dermatitis in North India. *Ind J Dermatol.* 1997;42:9-13.
9. Dhar S, Kanwar AJ. Atopic diathesis. *Ind J Dermatol.* 1996;13:81-2.
10. Kelleher MM, Dunn-Galvin A, Gray C, et al. Skin barrier impairment at birth predicts food allergy at 2 years of age. *J Allergy Clin Immunol.* 2016;137:1111-6.
11. Yashida K, Kubo A, Fujita H, et al. Distinct behavior of human Langerhans cells and inflammatory dendritic epidermal cells at tight junctions in patients with atopic dermatitis. *J Allergy Clin Immunol.* 2014;134:856-64.
12. Nakamura T, Hirasawa Y, Takai T, et al. Reduction of skin barrier function by proteolytic activity of a recombinant HDM allergen Der f I. *J Investigat Dermatol.* 2006;126:2719-23.
13. Nilsson L, Björkstén B, Hattevig G, et al. Season of birth as predictor of atopic manifestation. *Arch Dis Child.* 1997;76:341-4.
14. Monthemery P, Nihlen U, Goran Lofdahl C, et al. Prevalence of self reported eczema in relation to living environment, socioeconomic status and respiratory symptoms associated in a questionnaire study. *BMC Dermatol.* 2003;3:4.
15. Yuva A, Shimizu T. Trends in the prevalence of atopic dermatitis in school children: Longitudinal study in Osaka Prefecture, Japan from 1985 to 1997. *Br J Dermatol.* 2001;145:966-73.
16. Flohr C, Mann C. New insights into the epidemiology of childhood atopic dermatitis. *Allergy.* 2014;69:3-16.
17. Dhar S. Atopic dermaitis in Indian Children. *The Child and the Newborn.* 2001;4:47-51.
18. Morgentern V, Zutavern A, Cyrys J, et al. Atopic diseases, allergic sensitization and exposure to traffic related air pollution in children. *Am J Respir Crit Care Med.* 2008;177:1331-37.
19. Kramer U, Sugiri D, Ranft U, et al. Eczema, respiratory allergens and traffic-related air pollution in birth cohorts from small town areas. *J Dermatol Sci.* 2009;56:99-105.
20. Kramer U, Lemmen CH, Behrendt H, et al. The effect of environmental tobacco smoke on eczema and allergic sensitization in children. *Br J Dermatol.* 2004;150:111-8.
21. Van Bever HP, Llanora G. Features of childhood atopic dermatitis. *Asian Pac J Allergy Immunol.* 2011;29:15-24.
22. Tan B, Weald D, Strickland I, et al. Double-blind controlled trial of effect of house dust-mite allergen avoidance on atopic dermatitis. *Lancet.* 1996;347:15-8.
23. Kramer U, Weidinger S, Darsow U, et al. Seasonality in symptom severity influenced by temperature or grass pollen: Results of a panel study in children with eczema. *J Invest Dermatol.* 2005;124:514-23.
24. Doumes J, Cheng S, Travier N, et al. Farm exposure in utero may protect from against asthma, hay fever and eczema. *Eur Respir J.* 2008;32:603-11.
25. Langan SM, Flohr C, Williams HC. The role of furry pets in eczema: A systematic review. *Arch Dermatol.* 2007;143:1570-7.

26. Schuttelaar ML, Kerkhof M, Jonkman MF, et al. Filaggrim mutations in the onset of eczema, sensitization, asthma, hay fever and the interaction with cat exposure. Allergy. 2009;64:1758-65.

27. Von Mutius E. Maternal farm exposure/ingestion of unpasteurized cow's milk and allergic disease. Curr Opin Gastroebterol. 2012;28:570-6.

28. Chen CM, Sausenthaler S, Bischof W, et al. Perinatal exposure to endodoxin and the development of eczema during the first 6 years of life. Clin Exp Dermatol. 2009;25:238-44.

29. Mcpherson T. Current understanding in pathogenesis of atopic dermatitis. *Indian J Dermatol.* 2016;61:649-55.

30. Ross-Hansen K, Menne T, Johansen JD, et al. Nickel reactivity and filaggrin null mutations-evaluation of the filaggrin by pass theory in a general population. *Contact Dermatitis.* 2011;64:24-31.

31. Hata M, Tokura Y, Takigawa M, et al. Assessment of epidermal barrier function by photoacoustic spectometry in relation to its importance in the pathogenesis of atopic dermatitis. *Lab Invest.* 2002;82:1451-61.

32. Uehara M, Sawai T. A longitudinal study of contact sensitivity in patients with atopic dermatitis. *Arch Dermatol.* 1989;125:366-68.

33. Jakasa I, de Jongh CM, Verberk MM, et al. Percutaneous penetration of sodium lauryl sulfate is increased in uninvolved skin of patients with atopic dermatitis compared with control subjects. *Br J Dermatol.* 2006;155:104-9.

34. Hamann LR, Bernard S, Hamann D, et al. Is there a risk causing hypoallergenic cosmetic pediatric products in the United States? *J Allergy Clin Immunol.* 2015;135:1070-71.

35. Thyssen JP, Johansen JD, Linnerberg A, et al. The association between null mutation in the filaggrin gene and contact sensitization to nickel and other chemicals in the general population. *Br J Dermatol.* 2010;162:1278-85.

36. Bruckley DA, Basketter DA, Kan-king Yu D, et al. Atopy and contact allergy to fragrance: Allergic reactions to the fragrance mix I (the Larsen mix). *Contact Dermatitis.* 2008;59:220-25.

37. Tsakok T, Mckeever TM, Yeo L, et al. Does early life exposure to antibiotics increase the risk of eczema? A systematic review. *Br J Dermatol.* 2013;169:983-91.

38. Dhar S, Parikh D, Ramamoorthy R, et al. Treatment guidelines for atopic dermatitis by ISPD task force 2016. *Indian J Paediatric Dermatol.* 2017;18:174-6.

39. Dhar S, Kanwar AJ, Kaur S, et al. Role of bacterial flora in the pathogenesis and management of atopic dermatitis. *Ind J Med Res.* 1992;95:234-38.

40. Nakatsuji T, Chen TH, Two AM, et al. Staphylococcal aureus exploits epidermal barrier defects in atopic dermatitis to trigger cytokine expression. *J Investgat Dermatol.* 2016;136(11):2192-200.

41. Ardern-Jones MR, Black AP, Bateman EA, et al. Bacterial superantigen facilitates epithelial presentation of allergen to T helper 2 cells. *Proc Natl Acad Sci U S A.* 2007;104:5557-62.

42. Lange L, Alter N, Keller T, et al. Sensitization to *Malassezia* in infants and children with atopic dermatitis: Prevalence and clinical characteristics. *Allergy.* 2008;63:486-7.

43. Mpairwe H, Webb EL, Muhangi L, et al. Antihelminthic treatment during pregnancy is associated with increased risk of infantile eczema; randomized-controlled trial results. *Pediatr Allergy Immunol.* 2011;22:305-12.

44. Dhar S, Srinivas SM. Food allergy in atopic dermatitis. *Indian J Dermatol.* 2016;61:645-68.

45. Dhar S, Malakar R, Banerjee R, et al. An uncontrolled open pilot study to assess the role of dietary eliminations in reducing the severity of atopic dermatitis in infants and children. *Indian J Dermatol.* 2009;54:183-5.

46. Bath-Hextall F, Delamere FM, Williams HC. Dietary exclusions for established atopic eczema. *Cochrane Database Syst Rev.* 2008;1:CD005203.

47. Dhar S, Saxena A. Evaluating of prick test in atopic dermatitis and chronic urticaria. *Indian J Dermatol.* 1995;42:148-51.

World Clin Dermatol. 2018;4(1):100-11.

Microbes and Atopic Dermatitis

[1,*]Vanya Narayan MD DNB, [2]Rashmi Sarkar MD MNAMS

[1]Department of Dermatology, Acharyashree Bhikshu Government Hospital
New Delhi, India
[2]Department of Dermatology, Maulana Azad Medical College and
Lok Nayak Hospital, New Delhi, India

ABSTRACT

Atopic dermatits patients are susceptible to microbial infections due to various inherent and acquired factors. Such factors, common microbes, their pathogenesis, comparison with the normal skin microbiota, and antibiotic resistance is discussed in detail in this article. It briefly discusses the isolation steps for *S.aureus*. It also provides an insight into the 'hygiene hypothesis' with its mechanisms.

INTRODUCTION

Atopic dermatitis (AD) is a chronic relapsing eczematous inflammatory skin disease, usually presents during early infancy and childhood (Figure 1), but can persist into or start in adulthood.[1-4] Both hereditary and environmental factors play a role in pathogenesis. Environmental factors like foods, house dust mite (HDM) allergens, secondary microbial infections, and stress interact with the susceptibility genes in AD, and induce the production of immunoglobulin E antibodies and activation of Th-2 cells. Chromosomal regions of linkage to the disease have been identified in genome scans of children with AD.[5,6] This review will highlight the microorganisms in AD and discuss the reasons for their colonization and mechanisms involved in the initiation and exacerbation of disease activity by microbial components and its treatment.

*Corresponding author
Email: drvanyanarayan@gmail.com

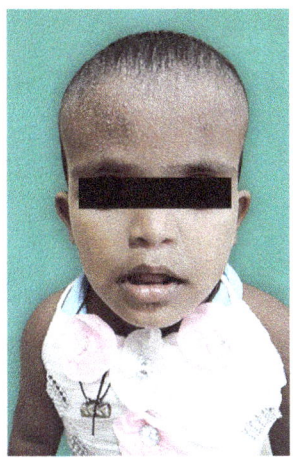

Figure 1: Facial involvement in atopic dermatitis in a toddler.

THE HYGIENE HYPOTHESIS[7-14]

The prevalence of atopy and associated allergic diseases is on the rise, partly due to decreased exposure to microbes in infancy that modulates the immune system. The decreased exposure may result from modern lifestyle factors such as reduction in family size, increase in hygiene and living standards and use of antibiotics. The relationship between decreased exposure to microbial antigens associated with a Western lifestyle and the increasing severity and prevalence of atopic diseases has become known as the "hygiene hypothesis." There are two hypotheses for the development of atopy as per "hygiene hypothesis." First states that innate immune cells, such as macrophages and dendritic cells, express pattern recognition receptors (PRRs) that recognize pathogen-associated molecular patterns (PAMPs) associated with microorganisms and on activation, such receptors induces a Th-1 type response. A lack of activation of innate immune cells by microbial antigen prevents the immune deviation from the Th-2 cytokine profile that predominates at birth to a Th-1 type profile and could explain the development of enhanced Th-2 cell responses to allergens.

As per second mechanism, lack of stimulation of dendritic cells (DCs) by non-pathogenic microorganisms in gut associated lymphoid tissue leads to reduced production of regulatory T cells [interleukin (IL)-10 producing]. Decreased production of regulatory T cells results in switching to atopic phenotype. In children with AD, *Clostridia* and *Staphylococcus aureus* numbers increased while *Enterococci* and *Bifidobacteria* were reduced in the gut. Selective probiotic bacteria induce IL-10-producing regulatory T cells *in vitro* by modulating dendritic cell function through DC-SIGN (dendritic cell-specific intercellular adhesion molecule 3-grabbing nonintegrin). This has led to the use of diet supplementation with *Lactobacillus* (as probiotics), even in the antenatal period, in both the prevention and treatment of AD.

COLONIZATION IN ATOPIC DERMATITIS

Patients with AD are highly susceptible to cutaneous bacterial, viral, and fungal infections (Table 1).[15]

The chief factors predisposing to infections in such cases are defective skin barrier (deficient filaggrin, involucrin, free fatty acids, ceramides),[16] deficient host defense molecules, increased adhesion, and defective clearance (especially with *Staphylococcus aureus*). Recently, a loss of function mutation in the *filaggrin* gene (chromosome 1, important for epidermal barrier) has been linked to childhood onset atopic dermatitis—providing a genetic basis for the disease.[17]

Staphylococcus aureus is the most common skin infection in AD.[18,19] Adhesion of *S. aureus* to the uppermost corneocytes is mediated by fibronectin and fibrinogen, components of extracellular matrix exposed as a result of Th-2 mediated injury to the barrier, specially by IL-4.[20,21] Defective barrier as a result of genetic mutations increases the transepidermal water loss and causes dryness which further increases the chances of colonization. Scratching further increases the adhesion by disrupting the barrier and releasing the cytokines that upregulate the expression of extracellular adhesins.[21] Further adhesion is supported by the ability of *S. aureus* to form a biofilm of hydrated matrix of polysaccharides and proteins.[22]

DEFECTIVE IMMUNE BARRIER

The first and nonspecific response of the human body to external aggressions is innate immune system. Components include an intact barrier with proper pH and microbiota, secretory elements, cell receptors such as pattern recognition receptors, and immune cells. Barrier is defective in AD both due to genetic factors, viz., filaggrin mutation and Th-2 mediated inflammation, and favors colonization by *S. aureus* as discussed above.

Table 1: Infections/Agents Associated with Atopic Dermatitis	
Bacteria	*Staphylococcus aureus* (most common)
Viruses	Warts (human papillomavirus), Kaposi varicelliform eruption or eczema herpeticum (herpes simplex virus 1), eczema vaccinatum (*Vaccinia virus*), coxsackie A virus, molluscum contagiosum
Fungi	*Trichophyton rubrum*

Secretory elements like antimicrobial peptides form part of this defense system, those which are triggered by inflammation of the skin—the defensins human β-defensin-2 (HBD-2) and HBD-3, and a cathelicidin, hCAP18/LL-37.[23] Human β-defensin-2 shows microbicidal activity against predominately gram-negative organisms like *Escherichia coli* and yeasts, but is relatively ineffective against gram-positive bacteria such as *S. aureus*. In contrast, HBD-3 and hCAP18/LL-37 are more potent that kill both gram-positive and gram-negative organisms and the yeast. Also, via the chemokine receptor CCR6, β-defensins can also act as chemoattractants for immature dendritic cells and memory T lymphocytes.[24] Reduced expression of HBD-2, HBD-3, and hCAP18/LL-37 has been shown in acute and chronic lesions of AD. Interleukin-4, mediator of Th-2 mediated immune response, has been shown to suppress the tumor necrosis factor (TNF)-α or interferon (IFN)-γ induced up-regulation of HBD-2 and HBD-3 in keratinocytes suggesting that the reduced levels of antimicrobial peptides may be explained by the predominance of Th-2 type cytokines in AD skin lesions.

The PRR comprises members of the toll-like receptors (TLRs), nucleotide-binding oligomerization domain-containing protein (NOD-like receptors or NLR), retinoic acid inducible gene, C-type lectin receptors (CLR) and peptidoglycan recognition proteins.[25] Toll-like receptors are well-known trans-membrane proteins capable of recognizing PAMPs and are expressed both by innate immune cells, such as DC, natural killer (NK), and macrophages, as well as adaptive immune cells, including T and B cells. Activation of TLR triggers the release of proinflammatory cytokines, therefore, modulating the immune response against pathogens. Toll-like receptor-2 is the receptor that recognizes lipopeptides from gram-positive bacteria, including *S. aureus*, suggesting that mutations of TLR2 may facilitate the susceptibility to *S. aureus*.[26] Nucleotidebinding oligomerization domain-containing protein receptors are intracellular receptors; NOD1 (also known as CARD4—caspase activation and recruitment domain 4) responds to gram-negative bacteria, and NOD2 recognizes a fragment common to all bacteria. NOD1 and NOD2 mutations are associated with AD.[27] NOD-like receptor proteins respond to ligands like DAMPs (damage-associated molecular patterns) and form a multiprotein complex termed inflammasome, which leads to the activation of caspase 1 and production of IL-1β and IL-18. Impaired NLRP3 expression may explain the chronicity of skin inflammation in AD. The C-type lectin receptors, viz., KACL (keratinocyte-associated C-type lectin), expressed by human keratinocytes, recognize sugars present in microorganisms and triggers cytolytic activity of NK cells and cytokine secretion. Although changes in the expression of CLRs have not been described in AD, atopic patients exhibit defective cytotoxicity of NK cells.[28]

Dendritic cells, the sentinels of the immune system, are antigen-presenting cells which express high levels of major histocompatibility complex class II

(HLA-DR) molecules, capable of recognizing and presenting antigens, leading to T cell activation.[29] There are two major DC subsets: CD11c+ myeloid DC (mDC) and CD123+ plasmacytoid DC (pDC); mDC (previously termed inflammatory dendritic epidermal cells or IDEC) are efficient in the uptake, processing, and presentation of foreign antigens, and under TLR stimulation, also induce secretion of TNF-α and proinflammatory cytokines, such as IL-12. These mDC provide an important link between aeroallergens and production of IgE. Immunoglobulin E has been shown to inhibit neutrophil adhesion, phagocytosis, and respiratory burst, which may affect clearance of microorganisms from the skin. Such mDC can be modulated by calcineurin inhibitors. Plasmacytoid DC are a source of antiviral type I IFNs (IFNα and IFNβ) and a reduction of these cells in AD skin facilitate infections such as eczema herpeticum.[30]

SKIN MICROBIOTA: NATURAL VERSUS IN ATOPIC DERMATITIS

Microbiota refers to the communities of microbes (bacteria, fungi, etc.) in an environment while the genes and genomes of microbiota as well as the products of microbiota and the host environment constitute the microbiome.[31] Skin microbiota varies depending on the body site and time. In general, bacterial diversity seems to be lowest in sebaceous sites with *Propionibacterium* being the dominant genus in such areas. *Staphylococcus* and *Corynebacterium spp*. are the most abundant organisms colonizing moist areas like popliteal and antecubital fossa.[32] The most diversity is seen in the dry areas like forearm, buttock, and various parts of the hand, with mixed representation from the phyla Actinobacteria, Proteobacteria, Firmicutes, and Bacteriodetes.[32]

Atopic dermatitis preferentially involves antecubital and popliteal regions, sites that harbor similar group of organisms and share distinct compositions of microbial communities (microbiome).[32] *Staphylococcus aureus* is inhibited by an acidic pH but skin occlusion results in an elevated pH, which favors the growth of *S. aureus* with mechanisms of increased adherence and penetration discussed previously. *Staphylococcus aureus* production of antibacterial compounds including bacteriocins and antimicrobial peptides contribute to relative decrease in *Streptococcus, Corynebacterium, and Propionicacterium species* observed during AD flares[33] (Table 2).

In exacerbations of AD, with *S. aureus* colonization, the number of *S. epidermidis* increases, suggesting a compensatory mechanism to control *S. aureus. Staphylococcus epidermidis* produces two antimicrobial peptides (phenol-soluble modulins γ and δ), which are selective for pathogens like *S. aureus* but do not combat *S. epidermidis*. Furthermore, small molecules secreted by *S. epidermidis* increase the expression of human β-defensin by human keratinocytes.

Table 2: Skin Microbiota—Natural Versus in Atopic Dermatitis	
Natural skin microbiota	**Atopic dermatitis skin microbiota**
Great diversity	Poor diversity
Bacteria: • *Staphylococcus epidermidis* • Coagulase negative *Staphylococcus* • Coryneforms (of the genera *Corynebacterium, Propionibacterium,* and *Brevibacterium*) • *Micrococcus*	• *Staphylococcus aureus* (predominantly), group A Streptococcus • Increased *Staphylococcus epidermidis* (compensatory mechanism) • Reduced other normal microbiota
Fungi: • *Malassezia* spp. (especially sebaceous areas) • Microscopic arthropods: *Demodex mites* (such as Demodex folliculorum and *Demodex brevis*) (esp. sebaceous areas)	
Viruses: • Not studied[34]	
High Shannon diversity	Low Shannon diversity

Another important bacteria with increased propensity of infections in AD is group A β-hemolytic *Streptococcus*. Its infection is often associated with severe AD. This may also lead to complications like post-streptococcal glomerulonephritis, hypertension, and post-reversible encephalopathy syndrome.

STAPHYLOCOCCUS AUREUS IN ATOPIC DERMATITIS

Staphylococcus aureus is usually classified as a transient pathogen, but in the anterior nares, it is considered as a normal component of the nasal microflora.[35,36] Colonization by *S. aureus* is not synonymous with infection.[37] The pathogenesis by *S. aureus* is largely mediated by the release of staphylococcal enterotoxins (SE), such as SEA, SEB, and toxic shock syndrome toxin-1, also referred to as "superantigens."[38] Superantigens cause nonspecific polyclonal activation of superantigen-specific T-cell receptor V families of T cells and upregulate cutaneous lymphocyte-associated antigen (CLA) expression by T cells via stimulation of IL-12 production, thus promoting their homing to the skin.[39] Superantigens also mediate effects on other cell types like eosinophils, Langerhans cells, macrophages, and keratinocytes. Eosinophils are recruited to the skin during AD flares by chemoattractants such as RANTES (regulated on activation, normal T expressed and secreted) and eotaxin, where they are activated and undergo degranulation and promote inflammation and tissue damage. Superantigens modulate the effector function of eosinophils by inhibiting eosinophil apoptosis, increasing expression of activation antigens (CD11b, CD45, CD54, and CD69), and enhanced cytokine activated oxidative burst, thereby triggering allergic inflammatory reactions.[40] They bind to HLA-DR on Langerhans cells and macrophages and stimulate them to produce IL-1, TNF-α, and/or IL-12 which increase CLA expression on T cells, thereby, facilitating the recruitment of CLA+ memory T cells to the skin. HLA-DR+ keratinocytes can also present superantigens to T cells which results in the activation of Th2 rather than Th1 cells as keratinocytes do not synthesize IL-12.

Many of the AD patients colonized with superantigen-secreting *S. aureus* produce IgE antibodies specific for the toxins found on their skin.[41] Basophils and mast cells from AD patients with antitoxin IgE antibodies release histamine on exposure to toxins, to which they have raised specific IgE antibody. Thus, toxins produced by *S. aureus* also exacerbate AD by activating mast cells, and basophils carrying the relevant antitoxin IgE antibody.

Staphylococcus aureus from the AD lesions can be identified by obtaining swab under all aseptic precautions and immediately inoculating into tubes of Mannitol-salt broth for further processing. After overnight incubation at 37°C, subcultures are made onto 10% sheep blood agar (Figure 2) and incubated again at 37°C and read the following day. Biochemical tests like tube coagulase test (Figure 3) aid in identification. Identification of isolates is accomplished by standard recommended techniques. Although *S. aureus* colonization is frequent in AD, methicillin-resistant *S. aureus* (MRSA) is still infrequent.[42,43] Methicillin resistance is due to the acquisition of a transferable deoxyribonucleic acid (DNA) element called staphylococcal cassette chromosome mec (SCCmec), a cassette (types I–V) carrying the mec*A* gene, encoding penicillin-binding protein (PBP) 2a.[44] Through site-specific recombination, the DNA element integrates

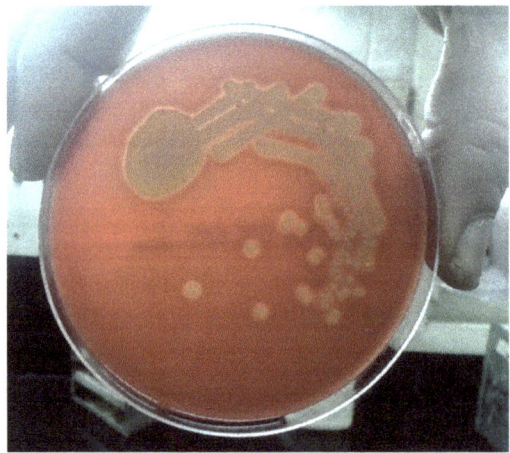

Figure 2: *Staphylococcus aureus* from atopic dermatitis lesions showing hemolytic colonies on blood agar.

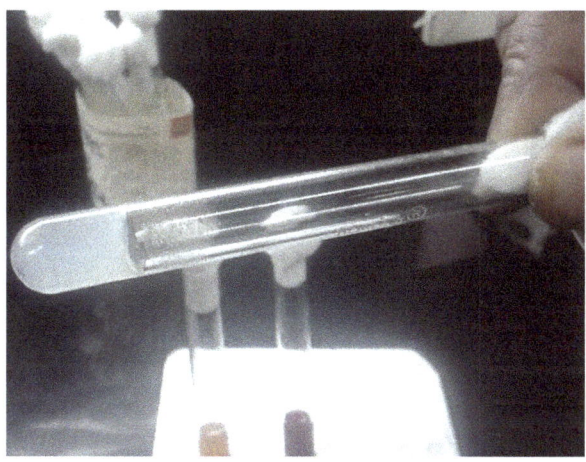

Figure 3: Positive tube coagulase test (suggestive of *Staphylococcus aureus*).

into the genome. Normally, β-lactam antibiotics bind to the PBPs in the cell wall, disrupt peptidoglycan layer synthesis, and kill the bacterium. However, β-lactam antibiotics cannot bind to PBP2a, allowing a bacterium containing the mec*A* gene to survive β-lactam killing. Since AD patients are rarely admitted to the hospital, MRSA isolates are commonly community-acquired, rather than hospital-acquired. Community-acquired-MRSA can carry a gene for PVL (Panton-Valentine toxin) which is shown to be associated with a severe infection. It has been shown that more than 50% of PVL positive MRSA are resistant to mupirocin which may alter the way such patients are being managed.[45] Data regarding vancomycin-intermediate and vancomycin-resistant *S. aureus* (VISA and VRSA, respectively) in AD is not available as of now.

Antibiotic susceptibility of *S. aureus* to the panel of antibiotics can be tested by the disc diffusion technique (Figure 4).

MALASSEZIA IN ATOPIC DERMATITIS

Malassezia (formerly known as *Pityrosporum orbiculare*/ovale) is part of the normal human skin flora and is most abundant at sites of high sebum production such as the scalp, chest, and back where it colonizes the stratum corneum. It regularly interacts with the skin immune system and hence, *Malassezia spp.*-specific IgG and IgM antibodies can be detected in healthy individuals. However, healthy individuals are usually not sensitized to *Malassezia spp.*, that is, they do not have IgE antibody to it. In 30–80% of AD patients, IgE and/or T cell reactivity to the fungus is present,[46] the reason for the high frequency of *Malassezia spp.*-

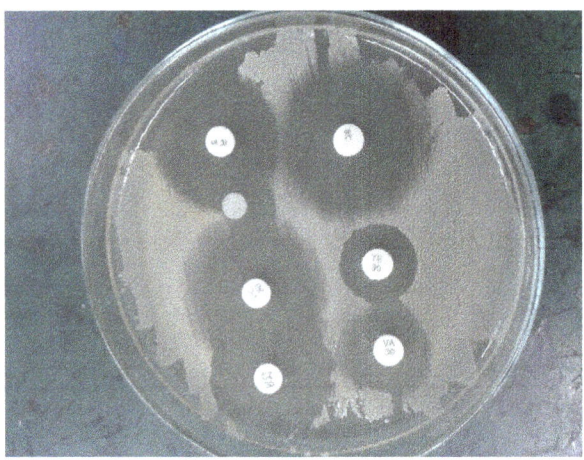

Figure 4: Testing antimicrobial susceptibility of *Staphylococcus aureus* using disc diffusion technique.

sensitization in AD patients is attributed to a combination of dysfunctional skin barrier, genetic background, and environmental factors. Patients with AD affecting mainly the head and neck region appear to be more likely to produce *Malassezia*-specific IgE antibodies, coinciding with the higher levels of yeast colonization in these areas than in patients with AD located elsewhere on the body. In children, there is lower frequency of *Malassezia spp.* sensitization compared to adults and the missing correlation between AD severity and *Malassezia* spp.-specific IgE can be attributed to the poor growth conditions for *Malassezia spp.* in children compared to adults. The lipid content of sebum, which is a prerequisite for skin colonization with most *Malassezia spp.* is low in children but rises during puberty. Accordingly, sensitization to *Malassezia spp.* seems to occur preferably in adulthood. As of now, 13 allergens from two *Malassezia species*, *M. furfur* and *M. sympodialis*, are listed in the official allergen nomenclature list. *Malassezia spp.* release more allergens in the less acidic environment of pH 6.0 that represents conditions of atopic skin and are internalized by the antigen presenting cells and causes maturation of dendritic cells and the production of proinflammatory and immunoregulatory cytokines, but not IL-12, thereby favoring the induction of a Th2 type response.[47] *Malassezia* also exerts proinflammatory effects by activation of the alternative complement pathway, and the stimulation of keratinocytes to produce inflammatory cytokines such as IL-6, IL-8, and TNF-α, which may contribute to its role in AD pathogenesis.[48] Toll-like receptors also mediate the communication between whole *Malassezia spp.* cells or their immunogenic proteins and human cells. It is known that particularly TLR2 recognizes components of yeast such as *Malassezia spp. Malassezia* also induces the expression of TLR2 and TLR4 on human keratinocytes which mediate the increased production of the antimicrobial peptide HBD2 and the chemokine CXLC8.[49] Also, mast cells of AD patients release increased amounts of IL-6 in response to *M. sympodialis* exposure.

VIRAL INFECTIONS IN ATOPIC DERMATITIS

Atopic dermatitis patients are also predisposed to viral skin infections, most common being caused by herpes simplex virus, eczema herpeticum. Other infections like eczema molluscatum is troublesome but not dangerous, eczema vaccinatum is rare but life-threatening. Genetic variants in the innate immune response may predispose AD patients to increased risk of viral skin infections. Such genetic variants include thymic stromal lymphopoietin, type I IFN (α, β, ω), type II IFN (γ), and molecular pathways that lead to the production of IFNs (IFN regulatory factor 2).[50]

CONCLUSION

Shannon diversity is lowered in atopic dermatitis with a predominance of *Staphylococcus aureus* and decreased number of other bacteria. The colonization of *S.aureus* is increased due to defective innate immunity combined with acquired factors and mere colonization does not contribute to infection. The pathogenesis is mediated by its superantigens. Atopic dermatitis patients are also prone to certain fungal and viral infections as mentioned.

Editor's Comment

This article highlights the microorganisms in atopic dermatitis, and discusses the reasons for their colonization, the mechanisms involved in the initiation and exacerbation of disease activity by microbial components, and its treatment. The concept of microbiome in atopic dermatitis and Shannon's diversity is discussed, this is very pertinent to causation and maintenance of atopic dermatitis in developing countries.

Rashmi Sarkar

REFERENCES

1. Spergel JM. Epidemiology of atopic dermatitis and atopic march in children. *Immunol Allergy Clin North Am.* 2010;30:269-80.
2. Friedmann PS, Ardern-Jones MR, Holden CA. Atopic dermatitis. In: Burns T, Breathnach S, Cox N, et al., editors. Rook's textbook of Dermatology. 8th ed. Oxford: Wiley-Blackwell; 2010.

3. Sarkar R, Kanwar AJ. Clinico-epidemiological profile and factors affecting severity of atopic dermatitis in north Indian children. *Indian J Dermatol.* 2004;49:117-22.
4. Spergel JM, Paller AS. Atopic dermatitis and the atopic march. *J Allergy Clin Immunol.* 2003;112:S128-39.
5. Lee YA, Wahn U, Kehrt R, et al. A major susceptibility locus for atopic dermatitis maps to chromosome 3q21. *Nat Genet.* 2000;26:470-3.
6. Cookson WO, Ubhi B, Lawrence R, et al. Genetic linkage of childhood atopic dermatitis to psoriasis susceptibility loci. *Nat Genet.* 2001;27:372-3.
7. Strachan DP. Hay fever, hygiene and household size. *Br Med.* 1989;299:1259-60.
8. Matricardi PM, Bonini S. High microbial turnover rate preventing atopy: A solution to inconsistencies impinging on the hygiene hypothesis? *Clin Exp Allergy.* 2000;30:1506-10.
9. Romagnani S. The increased prevalence of allergy and the hygiene hypothesis: Missing immune deviation, reduced immune suppression, or both? *Immunology.* 2004;112:352-63.
10. Bjorksten B, Sepp E, Julge K, et al. Allergic development and the intestinal micro-flora during the first year of life. *J Allergy Clin Immunol.* 2001;108:516-20.
11. Flohr C, Pascoe D, Williams HC. Atopic dermatitis and the 'hygiene hypothesis': Too clean to be true? *Br J Dermatol.* 2005;152:202-16.
12. Majamaa H, Isolauri E. Probiotics: A novel approach in the management of food allergy. *J Allergy Clin Immunol.* 1997;99:179-85.
13. Smits HH, Engering A, van der Kleij D, et al. Selective probiotic bacteria induce IL-10-producing regulatory T cells in vitro by modulating dendritic cell function through dendritic cell-specific intercellular adhesion molecule 3-grabbing nonintegrin. *J Allergy Clin Immunol.* 2005;115:1260-7.
14. Baker BS. The role of microorganisms in atopic dermatitis. *Clin Exp Immunol.* 2006;144:1-9.
15. Lubbe J. Secondary infections in patients with atopic dermatitis. *Am J Clin Dermatol.* 2003;4:641-54.
16. Elias PM, Hatano Y, Williams M. Basis for the barrier abnormality in atopic dermatitis: Outside-inside-outside pathogenic mechanisms. *J Allergy Clin Immunol.* 2008;121:1337-43.
17. Stemmler S, Parwez Q, Petrasch-Parwez E, et al. Two common loss-of-function mutations within the filaggrin gene predispose for early onset of atopic dermatitis. *J Invest Dermatol.* 2007;127:722-4.
18. Leyden JJ, Marples RR, Kligman AM. Staphylococcus aureus in the lesions of atopic dermatitis. *Br J Dermatol.* 1974;90:525-30.
19. Ring J, Abeck D, Neuber K. Atopic eczema: role of microorganisms on the skin surface. *Allergy.* 1992;47:265-9.
20. Cho SH, Strickland I, Tomkinson A, et al. Preferential binding of Staphylococcus aureus to skin sites of Th2-mediated inflammation in a murine model. *J Invest Dermatol.* 2001;116:658-63.
21. Cho SH, Strickland I, Boguniewicz M, et al. Fibronectin and fibrinogen contribute to the enhanced binding of Staphylococcus aureus to atopic skin. *J Allergy Clin Immunol.* 2001;108:269-74.
22. Akiyama H, Hamada T, Huh WK, et al. Confocal laser scanning microscopic observation of glycocalyx production by *Staphylococcus aureus* in skin lesions of bullous impetigo, atopic dermatitis and pemphigus foliaceus. *Br J Dermatol. 2003*;148:526-32.
23. Gallo RL, Murakami M, Ohtake T, et al. Biology and clinical relevance of naturally occurring antimicrobial peptides. *J Allergy Clin Immunol.* 2002;110:823-31.
24. Yang D, Chertov O, Bykovskaia SN, et al. Beta-defensins: Linking innate and adaptive immunity through dendritic and T cell CCR6. *Science.* 1999;286:525-8.
25. Kumagai Y, Akira S. Identification and functions of pattern-recognition receptors. *J Allergy Clin Immunol.* 2010;125:985-92.
26. Kuo IH, Carpenter-Mendini A, Yoshida T, et al. Activation of epidermal toll-like receptor 2 enhances tight junction function: implications for atopic dermatitis and skin barrier repair. *J Invest Dermatol.* 2013;133:988-98.
27. Weidinger S, Klopp N, Rümmler L, et al. Association of CARD15 polymorphisms with atopy-related traits in a population based cohort of Caucasian adults. *Clin Exp Allergy.* 2005;35:866-72.

28. Luci C, Gaudy-Marqueste C, Rouzaire P, et al. Peripheral natural killer cells exhibit qualitative and quantitative changes in patients with psoriasis and atopic dermatitis. *Br J Dermatol*. 2012;166:789-96.
29. Vittorakis S, Samitas K, Tousa S, et al. Circulating conventional and plasmacytoid dendritic cell subsets display distinct kinetics during in vivo repeated allergen skin challenges in atopic subjects. *Biomed Res Int*. 2014;2014:231036.
30. Zaniboni MC, Samorano LP, Orfali RL, et al. Skin barrier in atopic dermatitis: Beyond filaggrin. *An Bras Dermatol*. 2016;91:472-8.
31. Whiteside SA, Razvi H, Dave S, et al. The microbiome of the urinary tract-a role beyond infection. *Nat Rev Urol*. 2015;12:81-90.
32. Grice EA, Kong HH, Conlan S, et al. Topographical and temporal diversity of the human skin microbiome. *Science*. 2009;324:1190-2.
33. Iwase T, Uehara Y, Shinji H, et al. Staphylococcus epidermidis esp inhibits S. aureus biofilm formation and nasal colonisation. *Nature*. 2010;465:346-9.
34. Grice EA, Segre JA. The skin microbiome. *Nat Rev Microbiol*. 2011;9:244-53.
35. Peacock SJ, de Silva I, Lowy FD. What determines nasal carriage of Staphylococcus aureus?. *Trends Microbiol*. 2001;9:605-10.
36. von Eiff C, Becker K, Machka K, et al. Nasal carriage as a source of Staphylococcus aureus bacteremia. Study Group. *N Engl J Med*. 2001;344:11-6.
37. Cogen AL, Nizet V, Gallo RL. Skin microbiota: A source of disease or defence? *Br J Dermatol*. 2008;158:442-55.
38. Proft T, Fraser JD. Bacterial superantigens. *Clin Exp Immunol*. 2003;133:299-306.
39. Leung DY, Gately M, Trumble A, et al. Bacterial superantigens induce T cell expression of the skin-selective homing receptor, the cutaneous lymphocyte associated antigen, via stimulation of interleukin 12 production. *J Exp Med*. 1995;181:747-53.
40. Wedi B, Wieczorek D, Stunkel T, et al. Staphylococcal exotoxins exert proinflammatory effects through inhibition of eosinophil apoptosis, increased surface antigen expression (CD11b, CD45, CD54, and CD69), and enhanced cytokine activated oxidative burst, thereby triggering allergic inflammatory reactions. *J Allergy Clin Immunol*. 2002;109:477-84.
41. Leung DY, Harbeck R, Bina P, et al. Presence of IgE antibodies to staphylococcal exotoxins on the skin of patients with atopic dermatitis. *J Clin Invest*. 1993;92:1374-80.
42. Suh L, Coffin S, Leckerman KH, et al. Methicillin-resistant Staphylococcus aureus colonisation in children with atopic dermatitis. *Pediatr Dermatol*. 2008;25:528-34.
43. Chung HJ, Jeon HS, Sung H, et al. Epidemiological characteristics of methicillin-resistant *Staphylococcus aureus* isolates from children with eczematous atopic dermatitis lesions. *J Clin Microbiol*. 2008;46:991-5.
44. Hiramatsu K, Cui L, Kuroda M, et al. The emergence and evolution of methicillin-resistant Staphylococcus aureus. *Trends Microbiol*. 2001;9:486-93.
45. Regev-Yochay G, Rubinstein E, Barzilai A, et al. Methicillin resistant Staphylococcus aureus in neonatal intensive care unit. *Emerg Infect Dis*. 2005;11:844-50.
46. Scheynius A, Johansson C, Buentke E, et al. Atopic eczema/dermatitis syndrome and Malassezia. *Int Arch Allergy Immunol*. 2002;127:161-9.
47. Buentke E, Scheynius A. Dendritic cells and fungi. *APMIS*. 2003;111:789-96.
48. Watnabe S, Kano R, Sato II, et al. The effects of Malassezia yeasts on cytokine production by human keratinocytes. *J Invest Dermatol*. 2001;116:769-73.
49. Glatz M, Bosshard PP, Hoetzenecker W, et al. The Role of Malassezia spp. in Atopic Dermatitis. *J Clin Med*. 2015;4:1217-28.
50. Ong PY, Leung DY. Bacterial and viral infections in atopic dermatitis: A comprehensive review. *Clin Rev Allergy Immunol*. 2016;51:329-37.

World Clin Dermatol. 2018;4(1):112-7.

Moisturizers in Atopic Dermatitis

Jaspriya Sandhu MD DNB, *Rashmi Sarkar MD MNAMS

Department of Dermatology, Venereology, and Leprology
Maulana Azad Medical College, New Delhi, India

ABSTRACT

Atopic dermatitis (AD) is a chronic inflammatory dermatosis characterized by dry skin and the "atopic itch." Moisturizers primarily fall into three broad categories—emollients, humectants, and occlusive. Natural moisturizing factors include amino acid such as pyrrolidone carboxylic acid, urocanic acid, inorganic salts, sugars, urea, and lactic acid. The most essential aspect of treating a patient of AD is diligent explanation of general measures. Moisturizers are the backbone of every prescription for AD and a thorough knowledge of formulations is crucial to effective management, after gentle pat drying of the skin, an emollient should be applied within 3 minutes on slightly wet skin.

INTRODUCTION

Atopic dermatitis (AD) is a chronic eczema characterized by a relapsing and remitting course. The primary defect lies in the faulty barrier function of the skin which leads to increased susceptibility to environmental allergens and thus a state of chronic inflammation in the skin. The genetic basis of the disease is the *FLG* gene coding filaggrin protein whose loss of function mutation leads to aberrant barrier function of the skin.[1] So vital is the barrier function of the skin that it has been called the "raison d'être" of the epidermis.[2]

The most essential aspect of treating a patient of AD is diligent explanation of general measures. Moisturizers are the backbone of every prescription for AD and a thorough knowledge of formulations is crucial to effective management.

*Corresponding author
Email: rashmisarkar@gmail.com

MOISTURIZERS

Dry skin results from a loss of intercellular lipids, i.e., the ceramides, cholesterol, and fatty acids that form the bilayers which causes impairment of water barrier function. When there is breach in stratum corneum and moisture content is less than 10%, it results in dry skin.[3]

Moisturizers primarily fall into three broad categories:

1. Emollients
2. Humectants
3. Occlusives.

Emollients

Emollients are derived from the Latin word *ēmollīre*, which means "to soften." Emollients are saturated and unsaturated hydrocarbons which hydrates and smoothens the skin. Emollients include stearic, linoleic, oleic, and lauric acid and fatty alcohols naturally found in palm oil, coconut oil, and other vegetable oils (Table 1). They smoothen the skin by filling the minute cracks and fissures between the cells of the stratum corneum.

Humectants

Humectants are hygroscopic compounds, i.e., they absorb water from the surrounding both from the dermis into epidermis as well as from the environment.[4] This increases the water content of the epidermis. Humectants are low molecular weight compounds like urea, lactic acid among others (Table 2).

Table 1: Emollients	
• Isostearyl alcohol	• Glyceryl stearate
• Isopropyl palmitate	• Propylene glycol
• Decyl oleate	• Dimethicone
• Castor oil	• Cyclomethicone
• Jojoba oil	• Isopropyl isostearate

Table 2: Humectants	
• Alpha hydroxy acids	• Sorbitol
• Hyaluronic acid	• Honey
• Glycerine	• Ammonium lactate
• Pantethol	• Propylene glycol
• Gelatine	• Butylene glycol

Table 3: Occlusives	
• Petrolatum	• Cetyl alcohol
• Liquid paraffin	• Cholesterol
• Squalene	• Beeswax
• Lanolin	• Mineral oil
• Stearic acid	

Table 4: Natural Moisturizing Factors[7]	
• Free amino acids	• Urea
• Lactates	• Phosphate
• Sugars, inorganic acids, peptides, other unidentified materials	• Magnesium
	• Potassium
• Ammonia: Uric acid, glucosamines, creatinine	• Sodium

Occlusives

Occlusives are substances that act by forming a physical barrier between the skin and environment and thus limit transepidermal water loss. They are inert compounds often derived from petroleum by-products that act as effective moisturizers especially in inflamed, oozy skin (Table 3).

Natural Moisturizing Factors

Ceramides are a family of waxy lipid molecules composed of sphingosine and fatty acids. These preparations are also now available in microvesicular emulsions.[5]

The term natural moisturizing factors (NMFs) was coined in the 1950s by Jacobi et al.[6] These are naturally occurring hygroscopic substances within the corneocytes. Natural moisturizing factors include amino acid such as pyrrolidone carboxylic acid, urocanic acid, inorganic salts, sugars, urea, and lactic acid (Table 4).

PATHOLOGY IN ATOPIC DERMATITIS

Filaggrin (37 kDa) is a protein found in the corneocytes derived from the precursor molecule profilaggrin located in the keratohyalin granules of the stratum granulosum. Filaggrin plays an important role in the formation of the cell envelope of the corneocytes, as it catalyzes the formation of disulphide bond. Filaggrin in turn continues to be degraded in the stratum corneum to form NMF. The NMF bound water is essential for hydration of the skin. A study by Mclean et al. showed that the filaggrin mutation is carried by 10% of the European population.[8] A loss of function of mutation of the filaggrin gene results in atopic eczema resulting in characteristic dry skin and impaired barrier function of the skin.[9]

BATHING AND MOISTURIZING FOR ATOPIC DERMATITIS

Hebra first proposed frequent bathing 3–4 times a day as supportive measure for eczema in the 19th century. It was in the mid-20th century that Scholtz first proposed that bathing causes dryness of the skin and advocated bathing avoidance and application of emollient.[10] Thus, the oft-repeated paradox "bathing dries the skin."

General measures need to be explained in detail to ensure compliance. Soaking of skin is recommended for short periods no longer than 10–15 minutes, with a nondrying soap or nonsoap cleanser. Most soaps are alkaline in pH, whereas the skin's normal pH is 4–5.5, syndet based soaps may be preferred as they match the pH of the skin. Hot water baths, bath oil, scented oils, and scrubs are best avoided. Water if left to dry on its own results in greater transepidermal water loss. Thus, after gentle pat drying of the skin, an emollient should be applied within 3 minutes on slightly wet skin. Wet-wrapping may be done during acute flares of the disease.

In a study it was found that in AD subjects, emollient alone yielded a significantly (p <0.05) greater mean hydration over 90 minutes than bathing with immediate emollient, bathing and delayed emollient, and bathing alone.[11]

Which Moisturizer Should Be Used?

- For routine care: Emollients are easy to use, nongreasy preparations that may be used for routine care immediately after bath
- During flare: Occlusives may be used as they do not contain any preservative and thus do not irritate the inflamed skin
- For excessively dry skin: Lotion formulations maybe avoided as they lead to loss of water due to evaporation.

How Much Moisturizer Is to Be Applied?

Patients as well as their caregivers need to be educated about the appropriate amount of moisturizer to be applied where the finger-tip unit chart maybe given to the patient.[12] Patients should be educated about their medications and treatment objectives using the SMART method, i.e., specific, measurable, attainable, relevant, and time-based goals that is used for patient education in chronic disease (Table 5).[13]

Table 5: SMART Goals for Patients with Atopic Dermatitis

- WHAT? The patient should know the name of two formulations and why he/she is using them
- WHY? To increase knowledge regarding the disease leading to better adherence to therapy
- WHEN? At the end of two weeks, patient should be able to verbalize the names of the medication and why he/she is using it

CONCLUSION

Atopic dermatitis is a chronic disease whose treatment should be patient centric rather than physician centric. Patient education about the correct usage of moisturizers goes a long way in aiding successful management of disease. Patient acceptability, disease activity as well as cost should be used as a guide while prescribing appropriate therapy.

A clear and succinct knowledge of various formulations and their optimum use is thus a useful resource in the dermatologist's armamentarium.

Editor's Comment

The most essential aspect of treating a patient of AD is diligent explanation of general measures. Moisturizers are the backbone of every prescription for atopic dermatitis, and a thorough knowledge of formulations is crucial to effective management. Both cheaper emollients, and those containing ceramides and natural moisturizing factors are discussed.

Rashmi Sarkar

REFERENCES

1. Palmer CN, Irvine AD, Terron-Kwiatkowski A, et al. Common loss-of-function variants of the epidermal barrier protein filaggrin are a major predisposing factor for atopic dermatitis. *Nat Genet.* 2006;38(4):441-6.
2. Madison KC. Barrier function of the skin: "La Raison d'Être" of the epidermis. *J Invest Dermatol.* 2003;121(2):231-41.
3. Lynde CW. Moisturizers: What they are and how they work. Skin Therapy Lett. 2001;6(13):3-5.
4. Sarkar R. Moisturizers. New Delhi: Jaypee Brothers Medical Publishers (P) Ltd.; 2017.
5. Zeichner JA, Del Rosso JQ. Multivesicular emulsion ceramide-containing moisturizers: An evaluation of their role in the management of common skin disorders. *J Clin Aesthet Dermatol.* 2016;9(12):26-32.
6. Jacobi O. About the mechanism of moisture regulation in the horny layer of the skin. *Proc Sci Sect Toilet Goods Assoc.* 1959;31:22-4.
7. Clar EJ. Pyrrolidone carboxylic acid and the skin [in French]. *Int J Cosmet Sci.* 1981;3(3):101-13.

8. McLean WH. The allergy gene: how a mutation in a skin protein revealed a link between eczema and asthma. *F1000 Med Rep.* 2011;3:2.
9. McLean WH. Filaggrin failure - from ichthyosis vulgaris to atopic eczema and beyond. *Br J Dermatol.* 2016;175 Suppl 2:4-7.
10. Scholtz JR. Management of atopic dermatitis: A preliminary report. *Calif Med.* 1964;100:103-5.
11. Chiang C, Eichenfield LF. Quantitative assessment of combination bathing and/or moisturizing regimens on skin hydration in atopic dermatitis. *Pediatr Dermatol.* 2009;26(3):273-8.
12. Long CC, Mills CM, Finlay AY. A practical guide to topical therapy in children. *Br J Dermatol.* 1998;138(2):293-6.
13. Giam YC, Hebert AA, Dizon MV, et al. A review on the role of moisturizers for atopic dermatitis. *Asia Pac Allergy.* 2016;6(2):120-8.

World Clin Dermatol. 2018;4(1):118-36.

Atopic Dermatitis in Developing Countries with Emphasis on India

*Isha Narang MD, Rashmi Sarkar MD MNAMS

Department of Dermatology, Venereology, and Leprology
Maulana Azad Medical College, New Delhi, India

ABSTRACT

Atopic dermatitis is a disease of infants and children which has been initially described in developed countries but the literature and experience from developing countries are enriching our knowledge of this disease and has revealed few of its unique features. Previously considered uncommon, there has been an increasing trend of the disease. The disease prevalence and course is influenced by various environmental factors. Also, in etiopathogenesis, the environmental factors play an important role. Atopic dermatitis also impacts adversely in the form of financial drain and increased psychological morbidity. Diagnosis remains largely clinical and variability in significance of minor clinical features have been found along with some unique features observed in this population. Therapeutic plan emphasizes on cost effective and indigenous therapies. Emollients in form of oils and topical corticosteroids are popular. Counseling of parents and overall health of the child adds to the efficacy of the management plan.

INTRODUCTION

Atopic dermatitis (AD) is well described in developed countries, but in the last few decades there has been a plethora of literature and studies that has added to our knowledge of AD especially from developing countries like India. These different and unique aspects will be discussed below.

*Corresponding author
Email: ishanarang.d1@gmail.com

EPIDEMIOLOGY

The epidemiological studies conducted in India are described in table 1. Most of them are hospital based studies indicating variable incidence in ranging from 0.24%[1] (0–18 years) to 0.42%[2] (0–14 years), which is lower than in the Western world. An increasing trend of AD, especially in urban population, minor, inconsistent sex differences, and mostly winter aggravation have been observed.

India's varied climatic conditions due to its geography, influence environmental factors which further influences AD, showing wide variation in its prevalence. Atopic dermatitis is commonly seen in hot-dry, wheat consuming north India and less frequently in cooler-wet, rice consuming south India (0.01%). One hospital-based study from western India shown a higher prevalence (4.27%).[3,4] The initial epidemiological studies on AD in India showed lower incidence and later age of onset of AD compared to Western countries.[5] Protective effect of breastfeeding, longer weaning, and introduction of top-feeds later in the diet which exposes the child from food allergies at a relatively older age, were considered to be attributes to later age of onset.[6] However, further studies have demonstrated an increased incidence of AD probably due to urbanization, decline in breastfeeding and earlier weaning, and food additives. Also, there is an increased awareness of the disease among physicians and parents, smaller family, and delineation from disorders like infantile seborrheic dermatitis leading to better case detection.[5] This is also attributed to the importance given to skin diseases and establishment of dermatology as specialty branch in India.[2,5]

MORBIDITY

A study by Mina et al. confirmed the significant association of AD with anxiety, depression, and suicidal ideations. Prevalence rates of moderate to severe grade of depression or anxiety was found to be 15% and 12%, respectively. Also, women were found to be having significantly higher depressive and anxiety symptoms than males probably due to the reason that women are more concerned regarding their physical appearance than men. The study showed that higher educational status leads to more awareness and concern regarding physical appearance leading to medical consultation. Suicidal ideation was reported by significant proportion of subjects (16%) in this study similar to other studies. The study also showed more of suicidal ideation in women in comparison to men though not significantly, which could be due to more propensities of women to be affected by stressor and psychological distress leading to pessimistic view regarding the future.[9]

In a study by Sarkar et al. to determine psychological disorders in Indian children with AD and their mothers, increased psychological disorders were observed despite the disease being of less severity in the country. Psychological

Table 1: Epidemiological Parameters Studied in Various Indian Studies

Study	Sample size	Burden (%)	Male:Female	Age of onset	Mean duration	Social class (%)	Seasonal aggravation (%)	H/O atopy Personal history (%)	Family history (%)	Both (%)	Others	Severity	Type (%)	Clinical features (%)
Sinha (1972)[6]	166 Inf: 40	I: 0.38	Inf: 2:1	Distribution (%) 0–3 m: 12.5 3–6 m: 17.5 6–9 m: 20 9–12 m: 35 1–2 y: 15	0–6 m (55%) 6 m to 1 y (30%) >12 m (15%)	Poor: 57.5 Middle: 35 Rich: 7.5	Autumn and Spring: 7.5 Winter: 2.5	–	96.6 BA: 73.3 AD: 20 AR: 3.3	–	–	–	–	Site Cheeks: 80% Forehead: 7.5% Scalp: 5% Ears: 1% Extensor legs: 2.5% Extensor forearms: 2.5%
Dhar and Kanwar (1998)[2]	672 Inf: 210 (31.25%) Ch: 462 (68.75%)	I: 0.42 Among pediatric dermatoses: 28.46	Inf: 2.13:1 Ch: 1.09:1	Mean Inf: 4.2 m Ch: 4.1 y Distribution (%) 0–3 m: 4.6 3–6 m: 34.5 6–9 m: 26.9 9–12 m: 19.9 1–3 y: 9.4 3–6 y: 2.5 6–9 y: 1.6 9–12 y: 1	Inf: 3.3 m Ch: 1.9 y	Rural: Inf: 35.7 Ch: 32 Urban: Inf: 64.29 Ch: 68	Winter: Inf: 67.14 Ch: 58 Summer: Inf: 23.36 Ch: 32.9 Spring: Inf: 9.5 Ch: 7.4	Atopy Inf: 0.09 Ch: 15.37	Atopy Inf: 36.19 Ch: 36.37	Atopy Ch: 7.36	H/o drug allergy: Inf: 0 Ch: 3.16	–	Inf AD: Ac: 52.12 SA: 23.35 Chr: 23.35 Follicular: 0.46 Ch: Ac: 28.79 SA: 23.38 Chr: 47.4 Follicular: 0.43	Site Inf: Face: 79 Flexors: 42 Extensors: 52.31 Flexors and extensors: 5.7 Ch: Face: 74.5 Flexors: 35.53 Extensors: 56.32 Flexors and extensors: 8.24 Juvenile plantar dermatoses: 6.28 Hand eczema: 13.64 Cradle cap (In): 95.24

Continued

Continued

Table 1: Epidemiological Parameters Studied in Various Indian Studies

Study	Sample size	Burden (%)	Male: Female	Age of onset	Mean duration	Social class (%)	Seasonal aggravation (%)	H/O atopy Personal history (%)	H/O atopy Family history (%)	Both (%)	Others	Severity	Type (%)	Clinical features (%)
Dhar et al. (2003)[7]	100	Prevalence: 0.55	1.3:1	Mean: 4.58 y Distribution (%) 0-3 m: 17 3-6 m: 8 6-12 m: 5 1-2 y: 23 2-3 y: 20 3 y: 27	–	–	Winter: 15 Summer: 40 Rainy: 12 None: 33	54 BA: 33 AR: 21	65 AD: 40 AR: 18 BA: 7	–	–	SCORAD Mi: 54 Mod: 27 Sev: 19	Ac:42 SA:41 Chr:17	Face: 20 Flexors: 39 Extensors: 38 Both: 3
Sarkar and Kanwar (2004)[5]	Inf: 26 (20.8%) Ch: 99 (79.2%)	Among pediatric dermatoses: 29.9	Inf: 2.25:1 Ch: 1.6:1	Mean Inf: 4.5 m Ch: 4 y Distribution (%) 0-3 m: 13.6 3-6 m: 14.4 6-9 m: 12 9-12 m: 15.2 1-3 y: 24 3-6 y: 15.2 6-9 y: 4.8 9-12 y: 0.8	Inf: 3 m Ch: 6 y	Rural: Inf: 23.1 Ch: 31.31 Urban: Inf: 76.9 Ch: 68.68 Socioeconomic High Inf: 30.7 Ch: 19.19 Middle Inf: 53.8 Ch: 57.57 Low Inf: 15.5 Ch: 23.23	Winter: 62 Summer: 17	Atopy Inf: 42.3 Ch: 35.35	Atopy Ch: 7.07	Atopy Ch: 2.02	BF 100% <6 m: 11.54 >6 m: 88.46 W: <6 m: 15.38 6 m to 1 y: 30.77 >1 y: 53.84	Inf: Mi: 30.8 Mod: 57.7 Sev: 11.5 Ch Mi: 44.44 Mod: 56.57 Sev: 3.03	Inf: Ac: 65.4 SA: 7.7 Chr: 26.9 Ch AD: Ac: 27.3 SA: 28.3 Chr: 44.4	Site Inf: Face: 80.8 Flexors: 15.4 Extensors: 26.9 Ch: Face: 66.7 Flexors: 45.4 Extensors: 37.4 Cradle cap in Inf: 92.3

Continued

121

Continued

Table 1: Epidemiological Parameters Studied in Various Indian Studies

Study	Sample size	Burden (%)	Male: Female	Age of onset	Mean duration	Social class (%)	Seasonal aggravation (%)	Personal history (%) H/O atopy	Family history (%)	Both (%)	Others	Severity	Type (%)	Clinical features (%)
Kumar et al. (2014)[8]	132 Inf: 29 (21.97%) Ch: 103 (78.03%)	P: 7.21	Overall: 1.3:1 Inf: 1.4:1 Ch: 1.157:1	Inf: 5.2 m Ch: 3.47 y Distribution (%) 0–1: 28.8 1–2: 30.3 2–3: 19.7 3–4: 7.6 4–5: 3 5–15: 10.6	–	Rural Inf: 65.5 Ch: 61.1 Urban Inf: 34.5 Ch: 38.9 Socioeconomic High: 25.8 Middle: 46.2 Low: 28	–	Atopy 43.18	Atopy 33.34	Atopy 12.1	–	Overall: Mild: 42.4 Mod: 44.7 Sev: 12.9 Inf Mi: 27.6 Mod:48.3 Sev:24.1	–	Face: 76.8
Sehgal et al. (2015)[1]	100	P: 0.98 I: 0.24	1.8:1	3.63 y	1.46 y	Rural: 30 Urban: 70	–	BA: 37 AR: 42	AD: 14 BA: 43	–	–	SASSAD: Mean: 38.46	–	Face: 25 Flexors: 45 Extensors: 30

Inf, infants; Ch, child; I, incidence; p, prevalence; m, month; y, years; Mi, mild; Mil, mild; mod, moderate; sev, severe; BF, breast feed; W, weaning; SCORAD, Scoring Atopic Dermatitis; SASSAD, Six Area, Six Sign Atopic Dermatitis; Ac, acute; SA, subacute; Chr, chronic.

morbidity in the patients and their family members was observed due to scratching, disturbed sleep, and stigma of visibly affected skin. Fewer psychological disturbances in their mothers were observed possibly due to stronger family system and social support, and a less severe form of disease. However, more mothers of children with AD were submissive and overprotective which could contribute to the psychological disorders, a more dependent self-image and maintenance of eczema in the children. However, overall the mothers appeared well adjusted socially. There was also a statistically significant excess of conduct disorders and low intelligence with behavior disorders in children with AD over that in controls. Hence, psychological dimensions of AD should be taken into account as a part of the entire management plan.[10]

In India, due to lack of sensitivity towards mental disorders, psychiatry consult for disorders like AD and associated depression, anxiety, etc. is seldom taken. This is reflected in the fact that fewer studies have been undertaken in evaluating psychiatric morbidity related to AD in India as this problem remains elusive amongst both physicians and patient with respect to AD. This hurdle in management of AD has to be bridged in future and the problem seen is just the tip of the iceberg. In the authors' opinion, basic counseling and psychiatric consult can be more cost-effective in improving quality of life of patients with AD than the use of other expensive modalities and biologics.

Cost

Atopic dermatitis poses an economic burden on the budgets of families with patients suffering from this disease as in India, in contrast to West, the treatment is mostly self-funded. Health insurance cover, especially for dermatologic diseases is practically nonexistent in India. To quantify the expenses, a study was conducted and the cost assessment questionnaire was specifically designed for this which had a provision for measuring direct, indirect, and provider costs. The direct cost was measured for the outpatient registration and follow up fee, cost of investigations, and cost of the drugs (oral and topical). The providers cost were obtained from hospital data and the indirect cost was calculated in terms of loss of earnings of the caregivers. The cost of care amounted to approximately $93 (₹6,235) for 6 months and the annual cost comes to approximately $179–194 (₹12,000–13,000), which is similar to that of chronic illnesses like diabetes mellitus and schizophrenia in India. This cost is even higher in severe grades of the disease. This study also brings out the fact that monthly income of an average Indian is approximately $60 (₹4,000) and the cost of treatment may drain 25% of the total earnings. Hence, AD causes a blow to finances in patients of developing countries.[11]

ETIOLOGY

Heredity

In most of the Indian studies (Table 2) and in a study by Dhar et al.,[12] low incidence of personal and family history of atopy has been demonstrated. This has been attributed to the fact that most of the studies include pediatric population

Table 2: Evaluation of Minor Clinical Features in Various Indian Studies

Study	Kanwar et al. (1991)[23]			Nagaraja et al. (1996)[19]			Sehgal et al. (2015)[1]
Sample size	50 cases (%)	50 controls (%)	Signif- icance	100 cases (%)	100 controls (%)	Signifi- cance	100 cases (%)
Xerosis	80	20	**	76	14	**	–
Ichthyosis/ palmar hyper- linearity/keratosis pilaris	-/54/46	-/20/12	-/*/**	4/23/33	1/4/11	NS/**/**	50
Early age at onset	74	26	**	73	–	–	–
Tendency toward cutaneous infections	62	26	**	36	4	**	–
Tendency toward nonspecific hand or foot dermatitis	42	18	**	12	0	**	–
Nipple eczema	8	0	NS	1	0	NS	20
Cheilitis	6	0	NS	3	0	NS	58
Recurrent conjunctivitis	4	2	NS	14	0	**	25
Dennie-Morgan infraorbital folds	82	54	**	63	27	**	–
Keratoconus	–	–	–	0	0	NS	–
Anterior subcap- sular cataracts	–	–	–	0	0	NS	–
Orbital darkening	32	8	**	12	2	*	58
Facial pallor/ facial erythema	14	0	*	26	6	**	–
Pityriasis alba	78	56	**	34	28	NS	20
Anterior neck folds	12	2	NS	6	1	NS	–
Itch when sweating	66	12	**	35	16	**	–

Continued

Continued

Table 2: Evaluation of Minor Clinical Features in Various Indian Studies						
Study	**Kanwar et al. (1991)[23]**			**Nagaraja et al. (1996)[19]**		**Sehgal et al. (2015)[1]**
Sample size	50 cases (%)	50 controls (%)	Signif- icance	100 cases (%)	100 controls (%)	Signifi- cance	100 cases (%)
Intolerance to wool or lipid solvents	28	6	**	41	9	**	–
Perifollicular accentuation	22	10	NS	39	21	*	–
Food intolerance	-	-	-	0	0	NS	72
Course influenced by environmental/ emotional factors	26	6	*	S: 15 W: 29	–	–	–
White dermog- raphism/delayed blanch	12	2	NS	40/64	4/7	**/**	–
Infra-auricuiar fissuring	14	0	**	8	0	*	–
Diffuse scaling of the scalp	32	8	**	50	11	**	–
Hertoghe sign	–	–	–	0	0	NS	

*p <0.05; **p <0.01; S, summer; W, winter; NS, not significant.

and some of the manifestations of atopy develop later in life. Hence, it is possible that less severe forms of AD are associated with lesser prevalence of family history. Although role of heredity is strongly established, no studies have been undertaken in India to evaluate these factors in light of the recent developments of genes implicated in barrier function (like fillagrin) and those involved in immune response.

Environmental Factors

Various studies undertaken in India highlight the importance of environmental factors like pollution, use of oil (see below), hygiene, temperature, allergens, humidity, food, and clothing in AD. Also, a comparison between the severity in Indian children born and brought up in the United Kingdom and United States and that of Indian children born and brought up in India showed significantly higher mean scores of severity in the ones born and brought up in United Kingdom and United States, which was 8.64 than the ones born and brought up in India which was 6.34.

Microbial Factors

Staphylococcus aureus

There is higher degree of colonization with *Staphylococcus aureus* on lesional and nonlesional skin. Tropical climate of India further promotes this as is evident from a study, where it was isolated from 110 /119 (92.4%) patients and methicillin resistant *S. aureus* (MRSA) from 30 (25.21%) patients. Patients with MRSA had significantly higher Eczema Area and Severity index score.[13]

A study in our department showed from the lesion, maximum isolation coagulase negative *Staphylococcus* (CoNS), followed by *S. aureus*. In the nares, no growth was seen in maximum cases, followed by CoNS, followed by SA (unpublished data).

Parasites

Allergic diseases are rare in regions with high helminth parasite exposure and common where helminth exposure is lacking.[14] Endemicity to parasitic infections in India explains the low allergy risk but the improvement in socioeconomic status, hygiene, and reduced exposure to parasites may be an explanation for increased burden of AD in India.

Inhalant Allergens and Food Allergens

Food and aeroallergens have a role in AD especially supported by environmental factors in India. The skin prick test (SPT) was positive in 77.8%, i.e., 66.7% to aeroallergens and 11.1% to both aeroallergens and food. The most common aeroallergen group to which positivity was seen was dust. Others were pollen, fungus, insects, and *Dermatophagoides farinae*. Agricultural practices promote wheat dust and cotton dust as common aeroallergens.[15]

Serum immunoglobulin (IgE) levels and specific IgE antibodies were elevated in 88% of the patients and 65% of the children under 10 years were positive mainly against apple and hazelnut. Others were wheat, egg white, milk, potato, carrot, and codfish. Hence, it would be worthwhile to include advice about diet in AD patients. Specific antibodies to inhalants were seen more frequently in the older age groups. The enzyme allergo sorbent test positivity for the presence of specific antibodies to various inhalants was grass pollen (44%), dust mite (32%), animal dander (24%), mugwort pollen (14%), and molds (8%). In a South Indian study, the most common allergens causing sensitization were house dust mite (65–70%), trees (52–56%), and cockroaches (39–53%).[16] This indicates that grass pollens and dust mites were the most common aeroallergens.[17]

DIAGNOSIS

The diagnosis of AD remains largely clinical based on Hanifin and Rajka's 4 major and 23 minor diagnostic criteria.[18] Indian studies in tune with Western ones have shown variation in specificity and sensitivity in these minor clinical features.[19] There has been variability in significance of minor clinical features in Indian studies. Palmar hyperlinearity (Figure 1), keratosis pilaris, Dennie-Morgan folds, periorbital darkening (Figure 2), diffuse scaling of the scalp, facial pallor/facial erythema, itch when sweating, and intolerance to wool or lipid solvents have been significant minor clinical features, whereas icthyosis, anterior neck folds, recurrent conjunctivitis, nipple-eczema, and cheilitis as nonsignificant features. Diffuse scaling of the scalp was present even after the hair-oiling practices in India (Table 3). A statistical advantage of positive and negative predictive value

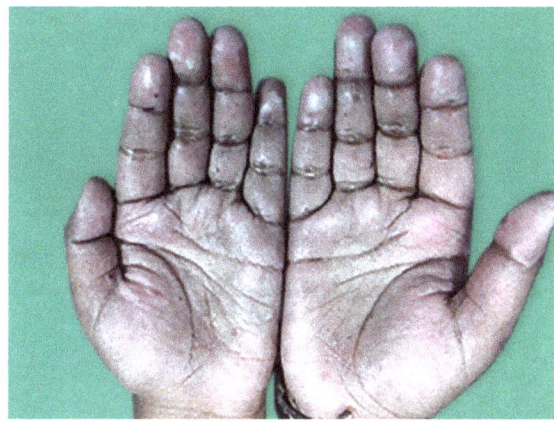

Figure 1: Palmoplantar hyperlinearity.

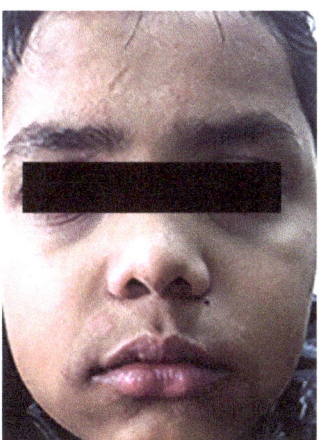

Figure 2: Periorbital hyperpigmentation with perioral dermatitis.

Table 3: Ocular Involvement in Atopic Dermatitis in Indian Studies

Study	Study population/ocular involvement	Recurrent conjunctivitis	Dennie-Morgan infraorbital folds	Keratoconus	Anterior subcapsular cataracts	Orbital darkening	Hertoghe sign	Lid	Conjunctiva	Lid or conjunctiva	Lid and conjunctiva
Kanwar et al. (1991)[23]	50 cases (%)	4	82	–	–	32	–	–	–	–	–
Nagaraja et al. (1996)[19]	100 cases (%)	14	63	0	0	12	0	–	–	–	–
Singh et al. (1997)	500 school children (%)	–	20	–	–	–	–	–	–	–	–
Dhar et al. (1998)[2]	672 cases (%)	–	–	–	–	–	–	4.98	–	–	–
Sarkar (2004)[5]	125 cases (%)	–	–	–	–	–	–	5.1	–	–	–
Kaujalgi et al. (2009)	100 cases (%)	–	26	0	0	–	–	18	16	43	9
Sehgal et al. (2015)[1]	100 cases (%)	25	–	–	–	–	–	–	–	–	–

of Hanifin and Rajka's criteria over the diagnostic criteria of United Kingdom working party was found in North Indian patients.[20]

For assessing the severity using the Rajka and Langeland grading in Indian patients, 41.25%, 50%, and 3.66% had mild, moderate, and severe forms of AD, respectively, with mean severity scores of 3.5, 5.7, and 8.3, respectively. A prolonged course and positive personal history of atopy was seen in moderate AD. This study showed milder disease in the North Indian children.[21] Also, children born of Indian parents living in the United Kingdom or United Sates showed higher mean severity scores than of those of parents living in India.[22] Milder disease here can be due to breastfeeding practices, vegetarian populations, and "hygiene hypothesis."

Morphology

In Indian patients, infantile AD presents as acute and childhood AD as chronic type.[2] Facial involvement is common in AD but only 20% had facial involvement in a study from the East in contrast to North India. This is probably due to pronged and severe winters.

Age of Onset

Infantile

It is acute in onset and starts at 4 months in India or younger, typically affecting face and scalp first (Figure 3). Cradle cap is a feature in a large Indian series.[5]

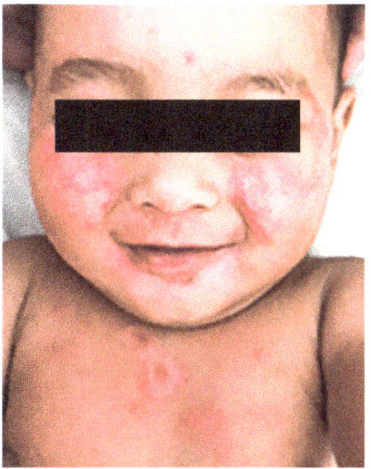

Figure 3: Infantile atopic dermatitis.

Childhood

It is chronic in onset presenting around 4 years of age, and overall of mild-moderate severity in India (Figure 4).[2] Other atypical features observed by the author in this population are follicular eczema, generalized darkness, infra-auricular fissures, retroauricular fissures, eyelid eczema, genital dermatitis, posterior thigh eczema, and juvenile plantar dermatosis.

Adult

The concept of adult-onset AD (onset >18 years), introduced by Bannister and Freeman,[24] was studied by Kanwar et al. in Indian patients. Of the adult patients referred to contact dermatitis, clinic over a period of 1 year, 18% fulfilled the Hannifin and Rajka criteria for AD. Dermatoses presented as hand eczema (52.77%), prurigo like lesions (30.5%), photosensitive dermatitis (22.2%), nipple dermatitis (22.2%), nummular eczema (16.7), lichenoid (11.1%), psoriasiform (5.55%), erythroderma (5.55%), eyelid dermatitis (25%), and periorificial dermatitis (13.8%). Clinical features in the elderly subjects (>65 years old) were same, except that flexural lichenification is uncommon and erythroderma was commonly seen. In India, airborne contact dermatitis (ABCD) or parthenium dermatitis is often indistinguishable from adult AD because of involvement of face, neck, and flexures. Patch testing is helpful in excluding the diagnosis of ABCD. Smoking is an important risk factor.[25]

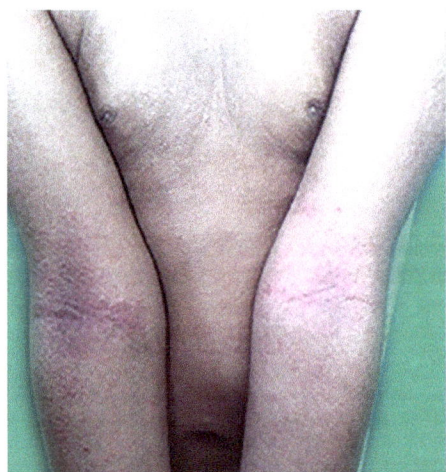

Figure 4: Flexural eczema.

Atopic Dermatitis and Eye

Less common ocular involvement and of low severity is observed in India atopics. Male predominance and 43% ocular involvement was found in a study.[26] Most of the Indian studies show involvement limited to only the lid and conjunctiva and none of the Indian studies (Table 4).

Table 4: Serum Immunoglobulin E Levels and Absolute Eosinophil Count in Atopic Disease in Various Indian Studies		
Study	**Immunoglobulin E levels (IU/mL)**	**Absolute eosinophil counts**
Sehgal et al. (2015)[1]	Mean: 1084.73	–
	Raised in 92% overall	
	New born: <1.5	
	Infants: <15	
	1–5 years: 100	
	6–9 years: 90	
	10–15: 92	
	>15: 50	
	Serum IgE levels and SASSAD score had highly significant positive correlation[1]	
Kumar et al. (2014)[8]	Mean: 1127.11	Mean: 1004.1
	Raised in 66%	Raised in: 69.7%
	• Mild: 389.28	Mean AEC in:
	• Moderate: 831.37	• Mild: 596.16
	• Severe: 1269.8	• Moderate: 850.17
		• Severe:1404.86
		AEC and SCORAD had positive correlation
Somani et al. (2008)[16]	Raised in 88%	–
	Specific IgE	
Dhar et al. (2005)[29]	278.2	624
	Serum IgE and SCORAD had positive correlation	AEC and SCORAD had positive correlation

SCORAD, Scoring Atopic Dermatitis; SASSAD, Six Area, Six Sign Atopic Dermatitis; AEC, absolute eosinophil counts; IgE, immunoglobulin E levels.

Atopic Dermatitis and Growth

In India, atopics growth velocities were lower especially in severe AD patients. Mean values for height and head circumferences were found to be significantly lower in girls probably due to more severe disease than boys. Preferential care and treatment to male children in contrast to females could contribute to the growth difference and severity of the disease.

Patch and Prick Test

Estimation of total serum IgE, specific radioallergosorbent tests, and SPT serves to ascertain atopy in an individual. Seventy five AD patients were patch tested using SPT allergens on the back, 47% of the patients showed positive reactions (*Parthenium*, 42%).[27] In another study where prick test was done in chronic allergic disorders among AD patients, maximum positivity was seen with *Dermatophagoides farinae*, pollen *Amaranthus spinosus*, grain dust wheat, and cotton mill dust; each comprising 22.22% of patients.[15] In a study to assess immunological response to *Parthenium hysterophorus* in Indian patients with *Parthenium* sensitive AD, 25 (35.7%) of 70 patients with AD had a positive SPT to *Parthenium*, compared to 3 (4.3%) of controls.[28] Hence, *Parthenium* appears to be an important aeroallergen in India along with dust mite. Absolute eosinophil counts and serum IgE levels were significantly higher in Indian patients and showed significant correlation with severity of the disease, with personal history of bronchial asthma and family history of atopy.[29] Patch and prick tests are not commonly performed as they are generally expensive and the experience of dermatologists in performing and analyzing these tests are mostly lacking.

DIFFERENTIAL DIAGNOSIS

Scabies and seborrheic dermatitis are two close differentials. Scabies can be superimposed on preexisting AD. Immunodeficiency states should be considered in infants with unusually severe disease. In Indian patients, improper hygiene, low socioeconomic status, and overcrowding leads to high prevalence of scabies. Also, poor nutrition, high prevalence of infectious diseases, and immunodeficiency states like human immunodeficiency virus/acquired immunodeficiency syndrome can complicate the disease course.

MANAGEMENT

In India and other developing countries, parents are seldom aware of this disease chronicity and its course. Time should be given so that parents are equipped with the information and means to take care of their children and know when to seek a physician's advice. This should be done in a simple and easy to understand way and in their own language. In India, specialist consult is seldom taken for skin diseases and in majority, the patients come in contact with pediatricians. There is a high chance of misdiagnosis and may even lead to enhanced side-effects due to prolonged usage of topical steroids. Complete immunization is important more as infectious diseases, malnutrition and overcrowding are issues which can aggravate the course of AD.

To get rid of crusts and eliminate bacterial contaminants, gently cleansing and bathing is essential. In India, bleach baths and Condy's baths (potassium permanganate) are cheap and easily available options. Oatmeal and sage baths are also popular. Saline compresses and potassium permanganate compresses, silver nitrate, or hydrogen peroxide can be used for oozy lesions. These also reduce colonization of *S. aureus* and further antibiotic use.

Emollients are foundations of AD management plan. Moisturizing depends on the season and is aggressive in winters than in summers and rainy seasons. Traditionally practiced oil massages utilize vegetable oils like safflower and sunflower oils, which offer many advantages like improving the skin barrier function, thermoregulation, and a positive effect on growth. However, a vigorous massage should be avoided. They are thought to be anti-inflammatory and antimicrobial, safe, and have lesser chances of allergic reactions than synthetic.[30] Beneficial effects of oils were also evaluated in a study comparing coconut oil versus mineral oil and placebo (powder) on growth where the massage with coconut oil, mineral oil, or powder was undertaken. Coconut oil massage proved to result in greater weight gain than mineral oil and powder. Those receiving coconut oil massages showed more length gain velocity than the powder group.[31] Evening primrose oil is also considered to be safe and effective medicine in management of AD.[32] Other essential oils like lavender and tea tree oil, honey, and aloe vera is also popular. Due to urbanization, working mothers, and diminishing large-family system, oiling practices are becoming less popular. Hence, there has been increase in prevalence and severity of AD. It was interesting to note healing properties of topical human breast milk as equal efficacy was seen against 1% hydrocortisone ointment.[33] Since it is a cheap and widely available resource, it can be advised to mothers in future in India.

A study advising a strict diet excluding milk products, nut products, egg products, selfish and prawns, brinjal, and soyabean for a period of 3 weeks was performed in India and significant reduction in severity scores was found.[34] It is a dilemma whether dietary restriction should be advised in India keeping in mind that a significant proportion of children are already nutritionally deficient.

Topical corticosteroids (TCs) are a first-line treatment in symptomatic patient. A cream formulation is preferred in hot and humid conditions of India avoiding complications like folliculitis. Topical tacrolimus ointment has been found safe and effective in Indian patients of moderate to severe AD and a statistically significant decrease in the modified Eczema Area Sensitivity Index was found. There was complete resolution to very good improvement in most of the patients and the drug was well tolerated.[35] Even though calcineurin inhibitors are more specific than TC and their side-effects are less, due to higher cost and its ointment preparation, TC still remain the mainstay in our setup.

Steroid-antibiotic combinations are still less popular. Combination of fluticasone and mupirocin led to a significant improvement in 90% of patients suggesting its efficacy, safety, and practicality in AD.[36] However, these regimens increase the overall cost.

There has been a good response to properly administered topical therapy and systemic treatment apart from antihistamine is not usually required. Oral steroids are given only in severe and recalcitrant disease. In an Indian study, oral erythromycin and cloxacillin given for 21 days in children with AD led to a significant improvement in eczema and pruritus and drop in the CFU/cm^2 of *S. aureus* suggesting that *S. aureus* aggravates the eczematous process and antibiotics decrease the severity and are useful in long term prognosis of the disease.[37]

Phototherapy is a second-line treatment. Its utility is restricted by availability and inconvenience of travelling to avail this treatment. It is mostly free of cost in selected government institutions; they are expensive in private sector.

For severe cases and acute exacerbations, systemic corticosteroids are rapidly effective but are used only for short course. Steroid sparing agents like azathioprine or phototherapy should be used in cases where prolonged systemic anti-inflammatory therapy is required. Methotrexate stands the test of time and is widely available immunosuppressive in the authors' setting as its cheap, easily available, and safe. Its safety in psoriasis in children is widely known in India but there are no studies for the same in AD from the authors.[38] As the disease is generally responsive to conventional treatment, there's a limited experience with cyclosporine, mycophenolate mofetil, and biologics.

CONCLUSION

Increasing urbanization and environmental factors have contributed to rise of AD in India. Establishment of dermatology as a speciality branch in India and increased interest of dermatologist has unfolded many unique aspects of the disease. Financial constraints and resource poor settings still restrict the therapy to indigenous methods and topical corticosteroids. Emphasis has been laid on overall nutritional and immunization status of children.

Editor's Comment

In developing countries, therapeutic plan emphasizes on cost effective and indigenous therapies to reduce the financial burden on the patient's family. Emollients in form of oils and topical corticosteroids are popular. Counseling the parents and overall health of the child adds to the efficacy of the management plan.

Rashmi Sarkar

REFERENCES

1. Sehgal V, Srivastava G, Aggarwal A, et al. Atopic dermatitis: A cross-sectional (descriptive) study of 100 cases. *Indian J Dermatol.* 2015;60(5):519.
2. Dhar S, Kanwar A. Epidemiology and clinical pattern of atopic dermatitis in a North Indian pediatric population. *Pediatr Dermatol.* 1998;15(5):347-51.
3. Karthikeyan K, Thappa DM, Jeevankumar B. Pattern of pediatric dermatoses in a referral center in South India. *Indian Pediatr.* 2004;41(4):373-7.
4. Jawade SA, Chugh VS, Gohil SK, et al. A clinico-etiological study of dermatoses in pediatric age group in tertiary health care center in South Gujarat Region. *Indian J Dermatol.* 2015;60(6):635.
5. Sarkar R, Kanwar A. Clinico-epidemiological profile and factors affecting severity of atopic dermatitis in north Indian children. *Indian J Dermatol.* 2004;49:117-22.
6. Sinha P. Clinical pattern of infantile atopic eczema in Bihar. *Indian J Dermatol Venereol Leprol.* 1972;37:179-84.
7. Dhar S, Mandal B, Ghosh A. Epidemiology and clinical pattern of atopic dermatitis in 100 children seen in a city hospital. *Indian J Dermatol Venereol Leprol.* 2002;47:202-4.
8. Kumar MK, Singh PK, Patel PK. Clinico-immunological profile and their correlation with severity of atopic dermatitis in Eastern Indian children. *J Nat Sci Biol Med.* 2014;5(1):95-100.
9. Mina S, Jabeen M, Singh S, et al. Gender differences in depression and anxiety among atopic dermatitis patients. *Indian J Dermatol.* 2015;60(2):211.
10. Sarkar R, Raj L, Kaur H, et al. Psychological disturbances in Indian children with atopic eczema. *J Dermatol.* 2004;31(6):448-54.
11. Handa S, Jain N, Narang T. Cost of care of atopic dermatitis in India. *Indian J Dermatol.* 2015;60(2):213.
12. Dhar S, Kanwar AJ. Personal and family history of 'atopy' in children with atopic dermatitis in north India. *Indian J Dermatol.* 1997;42:9-13.
13. Jagadeesan S, Kurien G, Divakaran MV, et al. Methicillin-resistant *Staphylococcus aureus* colonization and disease severity in atopic dermatitis: A cross-sectional study from South India. *Indian J Dermatol Venereol Leprol.* 2014;80(3):229-34.
14. Flohr C, Quinnell RJ, Britton J. Do helminth parasites protect against atopy and allergic disease? *Clin Exp Allergy.* 2009;39(1):20-32.
15. Bains P, Dogra A. Skin prick test in patients with chronic allergic skin disorders. *Indian J Dermatol.* 2015;60(2):159-64.
16. Mahesh PA, Kummeling I, Amrutha DH, et al. Effect of area of residence on patterns of aeroallergen sensitization in atopic patients. *Am J Rhinol Allergy.* 2010;24(5):e98-103.
17. Somani VK. A study of allergen-specific IgE antibodies in Indian patients of atopic dermatitis. *Indian J Dermatol Venereol Leprol.* 2008;74(2):100-4.

18. Hanifin J, Rajka R. Diagnostic features of atopic dermatitis. *Acta Derm Venereol Suppl (Stockh).* 1980(92 (Suppl. 144):44-7.

19. Nagaraja, Kanwar AJ, Dhar S, et al. Frequency and significance of minor clinical features in various age-related subgroups of atopic dermatitis in children. *Pediatr Dermatol.* 1996;13(1):10-3.

20. De D, Kanwar AJ, Handa S. Comparative efficacy of Hanifin and Rajka's criteria and the UK working party's diagnostic criteria in diagnosis of atopic dermatitis in a hospital setting in North India. *J Eur Acad Dermatol Venereol.* 2006;20(7):853-9.

21. Dhar S, Kanwar A. Grading of severity of atopic dermatitis in north Indian children. *Indian J Dermatol Venereol Leprol.* 1995;40:67-72.

22. Dhar S, Banerjee R, Dutta A, et al. Comparison between the severity of atopic dermatitis in Indian Children born and brought up in UK and USA and that of Indian children born and brought up in India. *Indian J Dermatol Venereol Leprol.* 2003;48:200-2.

23. Kanwar AJ, Dhar S, Kaur S. Evaluation of minor clinical features of atopic dermatitis. *Pediatr Dermatol.* 1991;8(2):114-6.

24. Bannister MJ, Freeman S. Adult-onset atopic dermatitis. *Australas J Dermatol.* 2000;41(4):225-8.

25. Kanwar AJ, Narang T. Adult onset atopic dermatitis: Under-recognized or under-reported? *Indian Dermatol Online J.* 2013;4(3):167-71.

26. Kaujalgi R, Handa S, Jain A, et al. Ocular abnormalities in atopic dermatitis in Indian patients. *Indian J Dermatol Venereol Leprol.* 2009;75(2):148-51.

27. Krupa Shankar D, Chakravarthi M. Atopic patch testing. 2008 September 1, 2008. Report No.: Contract No.: 5.

28. Kumar S, Khandpu S, Rao DN, et al. Immunological response to *Parthenium hysterophorus* in Indian patients with *Parthenium* sensitive atopic dermatitis. *Immunol Invest.* 2012;41(1):75-86.

29. Dhar S, Malakar R, Chattopadhyay S, et al. Correlation of the severity of atopic dermatitis with absolute eosinophil counts in peripheral blood and serum IgE levels. *Indian J Dermatol Venereol Leprol.* 2005;71:246-9.

30. Dhar S, Banerjee R, Malakar R. Oil massage in babies: Indian perspectives. *Indian J Paediatr Dermatol.* 2013;14(1):1-3.

31. Sankaranarayanan K, Mondkar JA, Chauhan MM, et al. Oil massage in neonates: An open randomized controlled study of coconut versus mineral oil. *Indian Pediatr.* 2005;42(9):877-84.

32. Senapati S, Banerjee S, Gangopadhyay D. Evening primrose oil is effective in atopic dermatitis: A randomized placebo-controlled trial. *Indian J Dermatol Venereol Leprol.* 2008;74(5):447-52.

33. Kasrae H, Amiri Farahani L, Yousefi P. Efficacy of topical application of human breast milk on atopic eczema healing among infants: A randomized clinical trial. *Int J Dermatol.* 2015;54(8):966-71.

34. Dhar S, Malakar R, Banerjee R, et al. An uncontrolled open pilot study to assess the role of dietary eliminations in reducing the severity of atopic dermatitis in infants and children. *Indian J Dermatol.* 2009;54(2):183-5.

35. Saple DG, Torsekar RG, Pawanarkar V, et al. Evaluation of the efficacy, safety and tolerability of Tacrolimus ointment in Indian patients of moderate to severe atopic dermatitis: A multicentric, open label, phase III study. *Indian J Dermatol Venereol Leprol.* 2003;69(6):396-400.

36. Khobragade KJ. Efficacy and safety of combination ointment "fluticasone propionate 0.005% plus mupirocin 2.0%" for the treatment of atopic dermatitis with clinical suspicion of secondary bacterial infection: An open label uncontrolled study. *Indian J Dermatol Venereol Leprol.* 2005;71(2):91-5.

37. Dhar S, Kanwar AJ, Kaur S, et al. Role of bacterial flora in the pathogenesis & management of atopic dermatitis. *Indian J Med Res.* 1992;95:234-8.

38. Kaur I, Dogra S, De D, et al. Systemic methotrexate treatment in childhood psoriasis: Further experience in 24 children from India. *Pediatr Dermatol.* 2008;25(2):184-8.

WORLD CLINICS
Statement of Purpose

The streams of medicine and surgery are evolving constantly at a rapid pace, creating a need for the healthcare professionals to continuously update their knowledge base and skills. This is necessary to offer their patients the best 'real world' treatment options based on current concepts, status, and trends, reflecting the achievements of evidence-based medicine. This pace of advances in medicine is a compelling reason for the physicians and surgeons to seek information through multiple resources such as journals, workshops and conferences.

WORLD CLINICS are periodicals of evidence-based reviews proposed as a source of comprehensive, state-of-the art reviews written by experts representing the global academia under the mentorship of an Editor-in-Chief. The comments by the 'Guest Editor' (or Editor-in-Chief) given at the end of each article/chapter would be representative of their clinical experience. Each issue of "WORLD CLINICS Dermatology" would focus on a single theme covering topics that are relevant to clinical understanding and decision-making. Each topic would be developed to reflect the current evidence, research, existing guidelines and recommendations as well the clinical experience of experts.

Objectives

- Provide up-to-date reviews on disease management, technique, procedure, or technology.
- Help enhance knowledge and skill for application in clinical practice.
- To aid use of evidence in decision-making for improved patient care.
- To help select best treatment options and overcome treatment challenges.

Target Readers

WORLD CLINICS are meant for practicing physicians, fellows, and postgraduate students, who plan to keep abreast with the current best-evidence clinical practices that are recommended and followed by experts globally.

Periodicity

WORLD CLINICS Dermatology will be released with a frequency of two issues per year.

Themes

Each subject area of WORLD CLINICS will cover themes on any of the following:

1. A disease or a disorder (e.g., Acne) OR
2. An organ or an anatomical region (e.g., Wrist, in WORLD CLINICS Orthopedics) OR
3. A technique or a treatment approach (e.g., Various methods for the treatment of CTEV, in WORLD CLINICS Orthopedics) OR
4. A special population group (e.g., Management of HIV infected pregnant patients in WORLD CLINICS Obstetrics and Gynecology) OR
5. A technology (e.g., 3D Ultrasound in diagnosis of gynecological abnormalities in WORLD CLINICS Obstetrics and Gynecology)

WORLD CLINICS
Manuscript Guidelines for Authors

General Guidelines

- Manuscripts must be typed in double-space including all text, references, tables, and figure legends, and should be sent in a single word file.
- For any copyright work, the necessary permissions must be obtained by the author and sent along with the manuscript. These permissions apply to any borrowed, modified, or adapted text, tables, or figures.
- For any production-quality artwork (images, illustrations, etc.) please see the guidelines under images.
- Acknowledgments or disclosures, if required, should be cited before the references.

Author Credits

- Should be in the first page.
- Each author's name, degree, academic or professional affiliation, city, and state (or country).
- E-mail address, mailing address, and telephone number of each co-author.
- If more than one author, mention the corresponding author.
- Please supply 4–6 keywords which will be used to optimize search results.

Subheads

The format for article's headings and subheadings is as follows:
'A' head: All caps, bold.
'B' head: Title case (upper/lower), bold.
'C' head: Title case (upper/lower), bold, italics.
'D' head: Title case (upper lower), normal, Roman.
'E' head: Sentence case (initial letter capital), italics, run in.

References

- References must be cited sequentially only at the end of the manuscript in the order as they appear in the text.
- Follow the Vancouver style for the references, using the Index Medicus abbreviations for journals that are indexed; if a journal is not indexed, use full name.
- If there are more than six authors, cite first six and add "et al."
  e.g., Lacasse Y, Selman M, Costabel U, Dalphin JC, Ando M, Morell F, et al. Clinical Diagnosis of Hypersensitivity Pneumonitis. *Am J Respir Crit Care Med*. 2003;168:952-8.

Images

- There is generally no restriction on number of boxes, tables, or images, but keep them to a minimum necessary.
- A maximum of two hand-drawn illustrations and maximum of two algorithms are allowed.
- Medium for delivery of photographs: Individual TIFF or JPEG files each at a resolution no lower than 300 dpi (118 pixels/cm) when viewed at 100 mm width.
- The images and illustrations can also be in full color.

www.ingramcontent.com/pod-product-compliance
Lightning Source LLC
Chambersburg PA
CBHW052135170526
45162CB00003B/23